Hindu Bioethics for the Twenty-first Century

SUNY series in Religious Studies

Harold Coward, editor

Hindu Bioethics for the Twenty-first Century

S. Cromwell Crawford

State University of New York Press

Published by
State University of New York Press, Albany

Printed in the United States of America

For information, address State University of New York Press,
90 State Street, Suite 700, Albany, NY 12207

Production by Kelli Williams
Marketing by Michael Campochiaro

Library of Congress Cataloging-in-Publication Data

Crawford, S. Cromwell.
Hindu bioethics for the twenty-first century / S. Cromwell Crawford.
p. cm. — (SUNY series in religious studies)
Includes bibliographical references and index.
ISBN 0-7914-5779-6 (alk. paper)
1. Bioethics–Religious aspects—Hinduism. 2. Medical ethics—Religious aspects—Hinduism. I. Title. II. Series.
QH332.C73 2003
174'.957—dc21 2002044796

10 9 8 7 6 5 4 3 2 1

To Matild

CONTENTS

ACKNOWLEDGMENTS

Thanks first to the Indian Council of Philosophic Research, Delhi, for selecting me to present the National Lectures for 1999 at four Indian universities on the subject of this volume.

Many ethicists have contributed to my thought, including Tom L. Beauchamp, Howard Brody, Daniel Callahan, James Childress, Werner Fornos, H. F. Haberman, Paul Jersild, Dale Johnson, Julius Lipner, Gerald James Larson, David R. Larson, B. Andrew Lustig, Jack W. Provonsha, James Rachels, Margaret and James Stutley, Robert M. Veatch, Mitchell G. Weiss, and Kenneth G. Zysk.

Among specialists in Indian medicine on whose writings I have liberally drawn, thanks go to L. S. Bhatnagar, Prakash N. Desai, G.P. Dubey, H. N. Gupta, Sudhir Kakar, Vasant Lad, K. R. Srikantha Murthy, A. Menon, P. Ray, M. Roy, P. V. Sharma, Shriram Sharma, R. N. Singh, Shrinivas Tilak and K. N. Udupa.

Colleagues at the University of Hawaii who have given me their support are Arindam Chakrabarti, Eliot Deutsch, Rama Nath Sharma, and Lee Siegel.

The International Religious Foundation has invited me to conferences to present papers on Indian medicine, thanks to Thomas G. Walsh and Frank F. Kaufmann.

Finally, *mahalo* to Harold Coward, editor of Series in Religious Studies, and Nancy Ellegate of the State University of New York Press for their confidence in this work.

INTRODUCTION

THE DISCIPLINE OF BIOETHICS

This is a philosophic study of Hindu bioethics. It represents a single Hindu model of the new discipline of bioethics, which is the application of ethical principles to the problems of medicine and biological research.

Bioethics is a product of the mid-1960s. Until that time, Hippocratic medical ethics served as the dominant Western model for some two thousand years. Its characteristic feature was paternalism. At all times the physician bore a profound sense of responsibility toward the patient's welfare, but this did not include the sharing of vital information, or acceding to the patient's wishes. Its fundamental premise was: the physician knows best. The Hippocratic tradition left its mark on modern medical ethics that, till a generation ago, comprised little more than a set of Victorian bedside manners and the doctor's duties to his professional fraternity. The thrust of paternalistic practice is capsulized in the dictum of the American Medical Association Code of 1847: "unite condescension with authority."[1]

Hippocratic medical ethics was obliged to abandon its paternalistic stance during the 1960s. In his essay, "Biomedical Ethics Today," Daniel Callahan recounts that Henry Beecher and a few colleagues at Harvard Medical School had observed that extensive biomedical research was being conducted on human subjects, often without their informed consent or without an objective assessment of the risks and benefits involved. Beecher blew the whistle on these activities, which led to the establishment of the Institutional Review Board system (1967) by the National Institutes of Health (NIH). "This was important as a public response to the moral problems of human subject research, and also as the first important signal to the medical community that in the future the public would have a role in monitoring and policing the ethical behavior of those with the biomedical research."[2]

Bioethics emerged as a discipline during the 1960s with the burgeoning of ethical dilemmas consequent upon the rise of two factors: (1) the explosion of medical knowledge and (2) new developments in medical technology, especially the technology of life support.

Following the wake of the deciphering of DNA's double-helix structure (1953), and the discovery of polio vaccine by Dr. Jonas Salk (1955), there emerged a phenomenal series of breakthroughs, such as the first heart transplant by Dr. Christian Barnard; speculations about genetic engineering; the routine use of dialysis; behavior modification by medical and surgical means; widespread use of respirators; the entry of the government into health care delivery through Medicare and Medicaid; and the work of Dr. Elizabeth Kubler-Ross with its stunning critique of excessive intrusions of medical technology for dying patients. All of these triumphs of modern medical knowledge and technology spawned a host of ethical dilemmas, not only for the medical community but also for American society at large; but as yet there was no scholarly organization independently able to tackle the new moral problems precipitated by these advances. Then, in 1968, as a result of the initiatives of Dr. Daniel Callahan, a philosopher, and Dr. Willard Gaylin, a psychiatrist, the Hastings Center was established in New York. The center is the oldest independent, nonpartisan, interdisciplinary research institute of its kind. Through studies, writings, and discussions, its goals are to explore ethical issues in the life sciences—particularly in biology and medicine, and also in the area of the environment. Equally noteworthy was the establishment of the Kennedy Center for Bioethics at Georgetown (1972), and the President's Commission on Biomedical Ethics (1983).

Advances in medical knowledge and technology continued into the 1970s and beyond. In 1972 British engineers invented the computer tomography (CAT) scanner, which assembles thousands of X-ray images into a highly detailed picture of the brain and also of the entire body. In 1978 Louise Brown, the world's first test-tube baby, was born in England. In 1979 the World Health Organization declared that smallpox had been eradicated. In 1981 doctors in San Francisco and New York reported the first cases of acquired immunodeficiency syndrome, or AIDS. In 1982 the U.S. Food and Drug Administration approved the first drug developed with recombinant-DNA technology, a form of human insulin. In 1995 surgeons at Duke University successfully transplanted hearts from genetically altered pigs into baboons, proving that cross-species operations can be done, and with the goal of giving pig hearts to humans. In 1997 Scottish embryologist Ian Wilmut reported that he and his colleagues at the Roslin Institute's genetic research facility in Edinburgh had cloned a sheep named Dolly from a mammary cell of a pregnant ewe—a procedure that made fiction become true, raising dreaded possibilities that stunned the world.

Today the modern medical revolution that began with Alexander Fleming's discovery of antibiotic penicillin in 1928, bravely marches on. Change has become almost addictive, a jolt to energy and creativity. Doctors vaporize tumors with laser rays, make babies in test tubes; and isolate memory cells. The most historic feat that changes medicine forever is the mapping of our DNA under the leadership of J. Craig Venter, CEO of Celera Genomics, and Francis Collins, director of NIH's Human Genome Research Institute. After a decade of heroic number crunching, groups led by these researchers deciphered essentially all the 3.1 billion biochemical "letters" of human DNA, the coded instructions for building and operating a fully functioning human.

Parallel to these advances in medical knowledge and technology, there have been other social developments that have precipitated the need for greater emphasis on ethics in medicine. These societal factors include:

- A heightened level of public awareness and education in matters of health
- The rise of peoples' participation in matters of their own health
- Civil rights and consumer groups that expect doctors to maintain high standards of treatment
- Legal and economic pressures on medical practice
- The emergence of diverse moral systems in society, and the need for greater awareness of the values and sentiments of non-Western religions, such as Islam, Buddhism, and Hinduism.

TRADITION AND THE BRAVE NEW WORLD OF BIOETHICS

Given the fact that the discipline of bioethics emerged from the scientific knowledge and technology of the late twentieth century, is it plausible to think that the dilemmas generated by these forces can be illuminated by religio-philosophic traditions that took shape in times that could not have imagined the possibility of bionic bodies, test-tube babies, organ transplants, and gene therapy?

First, it must be clearly understood that bioethics is only a special type of ethics to the extent that it has reference to a specific sphere of facts, namely medicine, and not because it incorporates some unique set of principles or methodology, which set it apart from traditional ethics. *The Encyclopedia of Bioethics* states: "Bioethics is not a new set of principles or maneuvers, but the *same old ethics being applied to a particular realm* of concerns."[3] (Italics supplied.) This being the case, no traditional form of ethics, be it Hindu, Christian, Muslim, or Buddhist, is disqualified from entering the field of bioethics just because it originated in a premodern, pretechnological era. As an example: *ahiṁsā* ("do no harm") is a cardinal virtue of most Hindu groups. This ancient moral rule is not challenged in medical ethics. Questions that do arise when *ahiṁsā* is applied in clinical situations are:

- Is the withdrawal of lifesaving therapy a case in which *ahiṁsā* is violated?
- Is the refusal to inititiate a life-support system necessarily contrary to the rule of *ahiṁsā*?
- Are we going against *ahiṁsā* when we allocate limited resources to another person with better chances for survival?

At no time does bioethics question the moral legitimacy of *ahiṁsā*, nor its philosophic presuppositions, grounded in Hindu tradition. It accepts the adage "Do not injure" as a rule of the old ethics. It only asks whether in a particular clinical setting, injury *actually* takes place. Furthermore, the entry of religion into the brave new world of medicine can work positively for medicine itself, and indeed is often an indispensable component.

First, religious traditions represent the collective wisdom generated by several thousand years of deep thinking on moral issues. They speak to our common humanity and address values that are unaffected by the march of time. They have developed universal ethical principles, such as the Golden Rule, which can be adapted to the latest situation. Dr. Willard Gaylin of the Hastings Center argues: "The genetic age will transform medicine, but the questions we pose are the eternal questions of justice, human rights, suffering and freedom. . . . While the metaphors of medicine are creative and captivating, the questions are for all of us to ponder."[4]

Second, through their affirmation of the transcendent dimension of human life, religions provide the element of sustainability in the bioethical enterprise, which serves as a necessary corrective to merely secular interests. Ethicist Jack W. Provonsha points out:

> Bioethics as an infant progeny of ethics has already largely taken over the house as infants are prone to do. Bioethicists are multiplying and new bioethics centers are appearing almost monthly. There is no question that these issues are fascinating. But the capacity for maintaining that interest through the perplexing years ahead is more likely to characterize those whose committment includes faith. So much about the answers to these questions is related to one's ultimate purposes as over against this-worldly professional goals.[5]

Third, the importance of religions for the bioethical enterprise comes out of their common origin in the human experience. People in all parts of the world and in every age face three fundamental problems: (1) how to maintain good health; (2) how to cure illnesses; and (3) how to delay death and reduce its attendant suffering. All three problems are as much concerns of religion as of medicine. Both players are *inescapably* brought into dialogue when confronted with beginning-of-life issues such as: procreation, genetics, abortion, contraception, fertilization, and birth. Religion and medicine are equally involved when we face end-of-life issues: soul, sanctity of life, quality of life, aging, autonomy, dignity, caring, suffering, pain, and dying.[6]

All these issues will be discussed in these pages. Given the unambiguous interface of religion and medicine, both historically and contemporaneously, it would be a grievous mistake to erect partitions between religion and medicine. What life has joined together, specialists and technocrats must not put asunder. There is indeed a duality of labor but a unity of spirit. As Jewish philosopher Abraham J. Heschel puts it: "The art of healing is the highest form of the imitation of God. . . . *Religion is not the assistant to medicine, but the secret of one's passion for medicine.*"[7] (Italics supplied.)

WHY THE HINDU POINT OF VIEW?

We have drawn attention to the fact that the new discipline of bioethics has many vexing topics to contend with: genetic engineering, total life support, fetal surgery, embryo transfer, to name a few. Added to the problems of the individual are the medical and health problems of society at large. As societal interrelationships become more complex, such medicine-related considerations as the food supply, housing, population control, and the ethics of the "lifeboat" have to be addressed. Under such mounting pressures, bioethics can use all the help it can get as it works its way into a new discipline. We propose to demonstrate that in this difficult venture, the Hindu tradition can prove a valuable ally. *In philosophical terms*, its diverse schools of thought, such as Sāṁkhya, Yoga, Nyāya, Vaiśeṣika, and Vedānta, are admirably suited to the demands of our pluralistic age. *In ethical terms*, the contextual structure of the Hindu approach gives it flexibility and adaptability, and invests it with the type of dilemmatic thinking that is required by contemporary bioethics in a world of rapid change. *In medical terms*, while Hinduism shares with all other faith traditions positive attitudes toward medicine and the healing arts, Hinduism is distinctive because it has evolved its own indigenous system of medicine that is based on medical manuals that comment directly on health issues.

Hindu bioethics flows from three basic principles of Hindu philosophy and religion:

1. The transcendent character of human life, expressed through the principles of the sanctity of life and quality of life.
2. The duty to preserve and guard individual and communal health.
3. The duty to rectify imbalances in the processes of nature and to correct and repair states that threaten life and well-being, both of humans and nonhumans.

Armed with these and other principles, we shall attempt to apply them consistently, comprehensively, and systematically to headline issues such as:

- Who tells a patient what information, in what manner, and how much?
- Who decides triage problems in patient selection and the allocation of scarce resources?
- Who resolves the issue of confidentiality when an adolescent consults a physician about contraception, about abortion, about drug use?
- When is a patient dead? When do physicians discontinue life-support mechanisms? How is the family involved?
- How should medics weigh the risks and benefits of new or experimental treatment?

The task of answering these questions is formidable. The road we have chosen is not only less traveled, but there are virtually no signs to give us directions, and a few that do appear point in all directions of the compass. The Hindu philosopher cannot help envy the Roman Catholic moral theologian who is left in no doubt in respect to issues such as contraception, abortion, surrogacy, and the like, because the mandates of the Vatican are clear, consistent, authoritative, and binding. But in Hinduism Varanasi is not the Vatican and a pandit is not a pope. Prakash N. Desai, a Hindu physician, accurately represents the present situation facing the Hindu bioethicist when he says:

> An organized body of knowledge for the ethical resolution of conflicts inherent in modern medicine is yet to be formulated in India. Given the diversity of belief and practice this task is overwhelming. But in the day-to-day life of Hindus, folk history is an important source of inspiration and moral examples. Ancient myths are renewed and reshaped, and as in the Hindu use of history, they become answers to philosophical and psychological dilemmas. It cannot be overemphasised that without an authoritative book or prophet to interpret ethical conduct for all Hindus at different times, the mythologies of ancestors serve as examples, and a single proper course does not exist.[8]

Desai goes on to explain that when people encounter some new conflict, they "make up a code of conduct by searching ancient lore for an appropriate example." As illustration, "abortion was legalized after legislative debates, and public argument was carried out mainly in secular newspapers and professional journals that borrowed heavily from ancient texts, both medical and religious, for supporting and opposing arguments."[9]

For the masses, whose illiteracy rate is as high as 75 percent, even this level of information is inaccessible, therefore they must "resort to minstrels, narrators of mythology, and folk theaters for the interpretation of such problems."

What role does the contemporary Hindu philosopher play in all of this?

A major irony here is that Hindu philosophers, notwithstanding certain assets of their traditions, have yet to leave their ivory towers and meet real challenges to their philosophies, not just in *logic* but in *life*. Jewish and Christian philosophers are deeply engaged in bioethical studies, but Hindu philosophers are still isolated in intellectual *asrams*. Why?

First, doing bioethics assumes a prior interest in ethics, which, judged by the number of Indian publications in this field, does not enjoy priority status. Even when ethics is discussed, it is pervasively through Western categories and modalities. The situation is even less complimentary when it comes to applied ethics. This lacuna is equally evident in the writings of Jain and Buddhist philosophers. In the Introduction to his work on *Buddhism and Bioethics*, Damien Keown expresses some despair: "Despite the contemporary importance of issues . . . there has been comparatively little discussion from a Buddhist perspective."[10]

Second, it must be acknowledged that the phenomenal growth of bioethics in the West has been the natural response to informational and technological developments. This situation has not arisen in India to the same degree, especially access to expensive medical technology, hence a similar urgency has not been felt.

Third, the philosopher doing bioethics must wear two hats—that of the philosopher and of the medic; yet the majority of philosophers in the Hindu area have not developed corresponding expertise in the facts, relationships, and concepts of the medical world to which the moral principles must be applied, and therefore they have not been able to engage in the bioethical dialogue.

The upshot of all of these factors is that in the present study we undertake a *maiden voyage* upon unchartered seas, but the perils of the passage will be more than compensated for by the thrill of discovery that this ancient tradition we call Hinduism is indeed *sanatana dharma*, even in the brave new world of bioethics.

Excitement for this project must not inflate its importance. If Hindu bioethics is a temple, we are merely laying its foundation stones, and like the work of all Hindu temples, the efforts of its earliest builders are made significant through the contributions of those who carry on the unfinished task.

Part One of this book presents foundations for an understanding of Hindu ethics and Hindu medicine. The ethical principles garnered from these investigations are then applied to diverse problems taken up in the sequel. Part Two deals with dilemmas pertaining to beginning and end-of-life issues.

PART ONE

FOUNDATIONS

CHAPTER 1

HINDU ETHICS

Satyam eva jayate nanritam.
Truth alone is victorious and not falsehood.

THE CONCEPT OF DHARMA

The Sanskrit word for ethics is *dharma* ("to hold"). It signifies that which upholds or embodies law, custom, and religion, and is analogous to the concept of 'Natural Law' in Christian ethics, though the idea of 'law' should not detract from its dynamic character. *Dharma* is activity, mobility, and is possessed of catalytic qualities. By contrast, *a-dharma* is stasis, stoppage, and therefore unnatural.

From the beginning of Indian civilization, the Indian mind has chiefly been preoccupied with the notion of *dharma*. K. N. Upadhyaya notes that "the persistence and intensity with which the inquiry into *dharma* has been pursued is mainly on account of the firm conviction of the Indian people that *dharma* constitutes the differentia of man," just as in Western philosophy, following Aristotle, rationality has been upheld as the mark that distinguishes humans from all other creatures.[1]

Notwithstanding this historic preoccupation with *dharma*, the Hindu scriptures do not have systematic discussions of moral doctrines, fashioned in the manner of Aristotelian or Thomistic models. At the same time Hindu scriptures are rich repositories of certain theoretical statements that define the shape of reality and the nature of things, along with prescriptive and practical sayings, aimed at the cultivation of moral behavior. The terminology in which these ideas and ideals are expressed is richly suggestive, making it possible to reconstruct these fertile fragments into models of systematic ethics.

The common scriptural ground on which the whole system of Hindu ethics is founded is the postulation of a *summum bonum* and the proper means to achieve it. This highest ideal is the state of liberation or *mokṣa*. In it a person finds self-fulfillment and deepest bliss. It is established on the metaphysical conviction of the oneness of Reality, which is attainable through direct experience. *Mokṣa* serves as the ultimate standard of right conduct. An act is of value or disvalue to the extent it either helps or hinders the attainment of freedom. Actions most distinctively oriented to *mokṣa* are those characterized by truth, non-violence, sacrifice, and renunciation.

At first glance the philosophical ideal of *mokṣa*, which calls for detachment and progressive resignation, appears antithetical to ethics, because ethics involves a person's active role in the world.

There is no doubt that the Hindu philosophical ideal transcends the ethical ideal, but, as with the rungs of a ladder, the higher and lower levels are connected and cannot function separately. Thus while Hinduism draws a sharp distinction between the spiritual and material, the eternal and the temporal, these dimensions of existence are not polarized but correlated within the inclusive concept of *dharma*. *Dharma* incorporates the metaphysical and practical wisdom of the Hindus.

The unity between philosophical wisdom and ethical excellence is clearly illustrated in the doctrine of *adhikāra*. This doctrine teaches that before a disciple can aspire after knowledge, he must first be morally qualified. The Upaniṣads are replete with references correlating *prajñā* or saving knowledge with moral practice. The Kaṭha Upaniṣad clealy states:

> Not he who has not ceased from bad conduct,
> Not he who is not tranquil, not he who is not composed,
> Not he who is not of peaceful mind
> Can obtain Him by intelligence (*prajñā*).[2]

Commenting on this verse, Rāmānuja explains that it "teaches that meditation, which should become more perfect day by day, cannot be accomplished without the devotee having broken with all evil. This is the indispensable condition of pleasing the Lord and winning His grace."[3]

The *adhikāra* doctrine underscores the intrinsic connection between rationality and morality. A truly rational person is bound to demonstrate qualities that are moral. In the pursuit of truth he or she is obligated to be free of bias, self-interest, and double standards. All of these are moral qualities. It follows that to be rational is to be moral, and just as a sound mind requires a sound body, a sound philosophy requires a sound ethics. Saksena says: "The moral and spiritual qualification of a philosopher is . . . a condition of his philosophizing properly. Passion or ethical failings cannot but distort the vision of even a philosopher. In fact, what is called intuition is not so much an independent faculty as a purity of the moral being of the knower which itself constitutes enlightenment."[4]

The moral discipline Hinduism enjoins upon the seeker after philosophical truth springs from a comprehensive ethic. Hindu ethics is a systematic progression from the Objective level to the Subjective level, culminating on the Superethical level. The first is the stage of Social Ethics; the second is the stage of Personal Ethics; and the third is the stage of the "Transcendental End."[5]

Objective Level: Social Ethics

In its objective aspect Hindu *dharma* is tridimensional. Social duties are classified as (1) *Āśrama-dharma;* (2) *Varṇa-dharma;* (3) *Sādhāraṇa-dharma.*

(1) Āśrama-dharma

The *āśrama* scheme provides the framework within which an individual may express the total needs of one's personality. These needs are incorporated within the doctrine of the four values of life or *puruṣārthas*, and are identified as: success *(artha);* passion *(kāma);* virtue *(dharma);* and self-perfection *(mokṣa).*

The *puruṣārtha* doctrine constitutes the psycho-moral basis of *āśrama-dharma.* It perceives human personality as a complex organism that is socially oriented. It recognizes an empirical side to life, represented by the first three *puruṣārthas*, having natural desires and social aims. Persons are conceived as naturally craving sex, and feeling the need for prosperity, power, and public good. The fourth *puruṣārtha* acknowledges a spiritual side to life marked by otherworldly hungers. Moreover, both sides are integrated within a holistic view of the person. Thus the *puruṣārtha* schema allows for no schism between desire and aspiration, or between the demands of the earth and of heaven. Both are good, when viewed relationally. True, the earth perishes, while heaven abides, but to treat the perishable as non-existing is to invite ruin. As the Upaniṣad declares: "In darkness are they who worship only the world, but in greater darkness they who worship the infinite alone. He who accepts both saves himself from death by the knowledge of the former and attains immortality by the knowledge of the latter."

Success is the first ideal worthy of pursuit. *Artha* is cognizant of the economic, social, and political needs of persons, and is especially important for a king. Through numerous passages wealth is praised, not only for its contribution to physical well-being, but also for its cultivation of social significance and political prestige. Wealth is said to transform a person of low social status to one of high status. Contrary to the adage, "Money is the root of all evil," it is said that "all virtues attach themselves to gold." However, there is nothing laissez-faire about *artha*; it must be regulated by *dharma*, and must express itself through liberality. "Let the rich satisfy the poor, and keep in view the long pathway. Riches come now to one, now to another, and like the wheels of cars are ever turning."[6]

Kāma is the second ideal every normal person must embrace. It refers to any pleasure derived from the five senses, including the sensuous enjoyment of art, music, literature, and especially sexual activity. Hindu religious and secular literature is replete with sexual allusions, symbolism, and undisguised eroticism. In the Middle Ages sexual intercourse was divinized to illustrate the wonder of creation, as figures of couples in close embrace were elaborately carved on temple walls. The celebration of sex reached its most exaggerated form with the introduction of ritual intercourse within certain religious sects. But, as historian A. L. Basham observes, this extreme form of sexual religiosity in the later Middle Ages was "only an expression of the vigorous sexuality which was to be found in Indian social life at all times." Here, too, *kāma* is not without limits: passion is good when it unites body and soul, and is regulated by dharma.

This brings us to the third value of life: *dharma*. It posits the moral nature and structure of the universe, because God is in it. The world is not just the evolution of an unconscious material force, creating and expressing itself in a world of increasing complexity and heterogeneity by its own unconscious dialectic. "It is a world of Divine and spiritual immanence with fullest reality of moral values and forces, because they flow from the power or Śakti of God."[8]

We have said that *artha* and *kāma* must be regulated by *dharma*. The rationale for this hierarchy of values is that whereas passion is born of inertia (*tamas guṅa*), and success is born of energy (*rajas guṅa*), the source of *dharma* is purity *(sattva guṅa)*—the highest of the three fundamental qualities of nature. By this criterion Manu enjoins that wealth and pleasure that are alien to righteousness must be discarded.[9]

Knowledge of one's own *dharma* or *sva-dharma*, as the Gītā puts it, is possible for the common person through a fourfold guide: (1) the Vedas; (2) the Smṛtis or expositions of Vedic wisdom; (3) the conduct of exemplary individuals; and (4) one's own conscience.[10]

The three *puruṣārthas* reviewed so far represent the ideals of the empirical life. They recognize and give balance to basic human needs. But higher than the desire of the empirical self are aspirations of the spiritual self. Maitreyī knew this well in her interrogation of Yājñavalkya. The old sage is forced to admit: "Of immortality . . . there is no hope through wealth."[11]

Immortality (*mokṣa*) is the fourth and highest *puruṣārtha*. It is the state of liberation wherein one's spiritual self comes fully into its own. Correctly pursued, *artha*, *kāma*, and *dharma* lead to *mokṣa*. Self-realization is not the negation of these mundane values, but their fulfillment.

Thus the doctrine of the four *puruṣārthas* presents Hindu ethics as a rich compendium of elements in life that less imaginative systems have deemed exclusive and antagonistic.

The structure of existence defined by the *puruṣārthas* calls for a correlative social organization through which human nature in all of its variegated forms is actualized. This is supplied in the *āśrama* scheme. Not only does this scheme channelize the individual's natural inclinations, it is a practical outlet for a sense of social obligations formalized in the ethical concept of the three debts (*ṛṇas*).

Before a person qualifies for *mokṣa*, it is obligatory to pay off vital debts. These are debts to one's teachers (*ṛṣi ṛṇa*), to ancestors (*pitṛ ṛṇa*), and to deities (*deva ṛṇa*). They are repaid through study, by begetting offspring, and through ritual performances. The notion of *debts* in the moral consciousness of the Hindu must be distinguished from the Western notion of *rights*. *Ṛṇa* is the by-product of a culture in which the whole web of life is seen as interdependent, and this elicits feelings of gratitude and responsibility.

Having explored the four ends of life and the three springs of social obligation, we pass on to the ethical organization in which the *puruṣārthas* are realized and the *ṛṇas* redeemed. The ancient Hindu philosophers were not content to theorize about life. They were practical enough to organize the life of the individual in such a way that he or she would have ample scope to find fulfillment in all areas of life. Modern Hindu philosophers should pay heed that the notion of applied ethics was a vital part of Upaniṣadic culture.

Āśrama-dharma enjoins that each individual pass through four stages in the quest for his true self. The *āśramas* are: (1) student (*brahmacārin*); (2) householder *(gṛhasthya)*; (3) forest-dweller *(vānaprastha)*; (4) hermit *(sannyāsin)*.

The student was expected to live at close quarters with his mentor, for the sake of training both mind and body. While the body was disciplined in continence, the mind was exercised in knowledge of the arts and sciences. In earliest times, women could enter *brahmacārya* and participate in Vedic studies, but the practice ceased when the pool of females entering society included persons deemed of lesser stock and custom.

The student was not expected to repress his desires for the opposite sex indefinitely, but was obliged to find fulfillment of his natural impulses in marriage. Marriage was upheld as a universal ideal, because it helped transform individuals with private interests and inclinations into companions commited in love to each other, and to future generations. Family solidarity included the living as well as members who had passed on.

When responsibilites to kith and kin are accomplished, as generations come and go, it is time to enter the third stage of life that leads to the forest and to a life of solitude and meditation. Social success has a point of diminishing returns, as the demands of the mind and the senses yield to the demands of the soul. A wife may join her husband if she shares his spiritual aspirations.

In the final stage, the path of life narrows and must be walked alone. The *sannyāsin* strives to free himself of all ego-consciousness that permits his unfettered Self to appear. Once a person realizes the Self, he or she becomes detached from all encumbrances associated with former notions of 'I' and 'mine.' Since detachment is fundamentally renunciation of ego consciousness, and not renunciation of the welfare of the world, a liberated person may continue to strive toward human well-being. Like the Buddha, moved by compassion, such a person may even eschew liberation from *saṁsāra*, in order to relieve the sorrow of creatures who suffer.

Thus the scheme of *āśrama dharma* answers the moral question of how a person should live by observing that there are distinct periods of life, each having diverse needs that call for diverse deeds. Morality is not monotone. Each stage is born of nature, and is therefore normal, necessary, and good. The moral life is less a matter of chronology, as of biology, physiology, and psychology. What is good for spring is not necessarily good for summer, and what is bad for autumn may be welcome in winter.

Varṇa-dharma

We now shift from the ethical organization of the individual, represented by *āśrama-dharma*, to the ethical organization of society, represented by *varṇa-dharma*. Both *dharmas* are coordinated, forming a composite system. Whereas the organization of *āśrama-dharma* approaches life from the side of nurture *(śrama)*, training it through successive stages; the organization of *varṇa-dharma* approaches life from the side of nature *(guṇa)*, defining the role of the individual in society by virtue of natural inclinations, tendencies, and innate dispositions.

The Sanskrit word *varṇa* literally means color. Originally it was connected with the class structure of the Vedic Āryan tribes. It is scientifically inaccurate to apply the meaning of "caste" to *varṇa*. Basham explains:

> There are only four *varṇas*. There never have been less than four or more than four. It is said that at the present time there are 3000 castes, and the number of castes is known to have risen, and perhaps has sometimes fallen, over the past 2000 years. Caste and *varṇa* are quite different institutions, different in origin, different in purpose, and different in function.[12]

Originally the class structure was devised to promote a functional harmony between the various segments of society. Society was conceived as constituting four distinct types. Brahmins belonged to the first type. They were the priest-teachers. Due to the assumed prevalence of *sattva guṇas* in their nature, they were deemed capable of living on an exalted plane of intellect and probity. The kṣatriyas belonged to the second type. They were the warrior-kings. Possessing a large portion of *rajas guṇa*, they demonstrated uncommon virility, and were primarily men of action. The vaiśyas belonged to the third type. They were traders and craftsmen. The dominance of *tamas guṇas* made them into persons of feeling. The śūdras belonged to the fourth type. Being manual laborers, it was assumed that they did not possess any of the traits found in the other classes.

Modern Hindus consider the rationale behind the original classification generally valid. Realistically speaking, all persons are not created equal. People differ in their gifts and graces. It is unwise and unproductive to put a round peg in a square hole. Mahatama Gandhi's comment on *varṇa-dharma* was: "It is a law of spiritual economics and has nothing to do with superiority and inferiority."[13]

However, it was not long before the original class structure was displaced by the law of heredity, and an ironclad caste system took on all the marks and trappings of superiority and inferiority in respect to food, clothing, language, ceremonials, social intercourse, marriage, and occupation.

The evils of the caste or *jāti*-system are too well known to bear repetition or reproach. It goes against the grain of Hindu *dharma* where only virtue counts. In the Mahābhārata, Yudhiṣṭhira teaches: "truth, charity, fortitude, good conduct, gentleness, austerity, and compassion—he in whom these are observed is a *brāhmaṇa*. If these marks exist in a *śūdra* and are not found in a twice-born, the *śūdra* is not a śūdra, nor the *brāhmaṇa* a *brāhmaṇa*."[14] In his study of the Bhagvadgītā, K. N. Upadhyaya notes that whereas the text accepts the caste ideal on religious, biological, and sociological grounds, it universalizes the orthodox concept of salvation to make it accessible to all persons, and refuses to categorize moral acts by hierarchical standards.[15]

Buddhism and Jainism were not alone in condemning the caste system; their opposition was taken up by Hindu sects such as Śaivas and Vaiṣṇavas. Modern reformers, such as Ram Mohan Roy (1772–1833) and Swami Dayananda (1824–1883), declared caste a departure from the Vedas; and Mahatama Gandhi (1869–1948) crusaded on behalf of India's outcastes (Untouchables), giving them the new designation of Harijans or sons of God.

Thus it was when India became a democratic republic in 1947, the abrogation of caste by her Constitution was not seen as being in conflict with the original spirit of Hindu social ethics.

Sādhāraṇa-dharma

In addition to *vishesha* or specific duties, objective ethics includes *sāṃānya* or 'generic' duties. Whereas the first is relative and conditional, the second is common and unconditional. The common duties (*sādhāraṇa-dharma*) are so named because they are independent of caste and station in life, and are binding upon humans as humans—all members of one community. As such, human rights precede communal rights. A brahmin wanting to make a sacrificial offering is not at liberty to acquire the object of sacrifice by stealth, for *asteya* or nonstealing is a universal duty. S. K. Maitra observes that notwithstanding the social degradation of the *śūdra*, the code of universal duties that are obligatory on persons as persons provide a certain amount of moral protection. He says, "These duties are to be observed by all alike, being the duties obligatory on everybody in his dealing with everybody else. They are thus to be observed not merely by the *shudras* but also by members of the higher caste."[16] What are these universal duties? Manu lists the following:

1. Steadfastness *(dhairya)*
2. Forgiveness *(kshama)*
3. Application *(dama)*
4. Non-Appropriation *(chouryabhava)*
5. Cleanliness *(shoucha)*
6. Repression of sensuous appetites *(indriya-nigraha)*
7. Wisdom *(dhi)*
8. Learning *(vidyā)*
9. Veracity *(satya)*
10. Restraint of anger *(akrodha)*[17]

It is apparent that the virtues in this list of universal duties are predominantly ascetical (steadfastness, application, and repression) and dianoetic (wisdom, learning, and veracity). Their end is self-culture, based on an ethic of autonomy. This harmonizes well with the law of karma that states that a person rises or falls by virtue of his or her own deeds. The emphasis on self-sufficiency is important, but we miss any reference to social service.

The element missing in Manu's list is partially compensated for in Praśastapāda's record of generic or *sāṃānya* duties. The humanitarian component comes through in the inclusion of duties such as *ahiṁsā* (refraining from injury to living beings), and *bhūtahitatva* (seeking the good of all creatures).

Objective ethics constitutes the first stage of Hindu *dharma*. On this stage morality is represented by social codes demanding external conformity. In psychological understanding, this is the stage of socialization and introjection. The voice of conscience is for the most part the interiorized voice of the group. The thrust of conscience is the sense of "must." The feel of conscience is driven by fear of punishment for duties not done.

Subjective Level: Personal Ethics

'Must' and 'Ought'

Hindu *dharma* is cognitively developmental. It teaches that one should progress from the 'must consciousness' to the 'ought consciousness.' This shift proceeds from a heightened awareness of the Self, which purifies the mind and issues in actions that are consistent with the true nature of the Self. This is the subjective stage of Hindu ethics, known as *Cittaśuddhi* or purification of the mind.

Subjective ethics is an advance over objective ethics, because virtues are superior to duties. Whereas duty is other-directed; virtue is inner-directed. Duty represents tribalistic morality; virtue represents individual morality. Duties are related to experiences of prohibition and fear, but virtues arise from feelings of preference and self-respect. Duty is ad hoc and specific, with reference to particular commandments, codes, and customs; virtue is generic and is expressive of fundamental orientations in life, such as the Golden Rule.

Thus, on the level of *Cittaśuddhi,* the purified mind internalizes the rules of objective morality, and transforms duty into virtue. You may continue to follow the old rules, but now it is not because you must, but because you ought. The quality of what you do, speak, and think is free, and this internal freedom is characterized by *vairāgya* or detachment. *Vairāgya* and virtue are two sides of the same coin. According to Vātsyāyana, virtue *(dharma)* has three forms, namely:

1. Virtues of the body—charity, helping the needy, social service
2. Virtues of speech—truthfulness, benevolence, gentleness, recitation of scriptures
3. Virtues of the mind—kindness, unworldliness, piety

Like virtue, vice is also threefold:

1. Vices of the body—cruelty, theft, sexual indulgence
2. Vices of speech—falsehood, harshness, scandal
3. Vices of the mind—hatred covetousness, unbelief

Transcendental Ethics

For all of its elevation of individual perfection, subjective ethics is not the highest level of spirituality. Like social ethics, personal ethics is not an end in itself but a means toward the ultimate end which is "the life absolute and transcendental." Here social morality and personal morality are reincarnated in a new light and "charged with absolute significance."

Maitra reminds us this precisely is the goal of Patañjali's Yoga, Śaṁkara's view of *mokṣa*, Rāmānuja's doctrine of *bhakti*, and the Buddha's understanding of *Nirvāṇa*. "All these agree in recognizing the transcendental as the limit of the empirical life, the timeless as the truth of all that is in time. This timeless, transcendental life is therefore the culminating stage of the spirit, the sphere of its consummation and fruition."[18]

This transcendental life is not a new acquisition, something given from above, like the Christian view of salvation. The self is already perfect, immortal, and free, but has been concealed through *māyā*. Through the veil of *māyā*, all one sees is the chrysalis, but when knowledge penetrates ignorance, the chrysalis is transformed into a butterfly. The transformation is a total experience, which reveals the essential nature of the soul as pure existence *(sat)*, pure consciousness *(cit)*, and pure bliss *(ánanda)*.

The transcendental level of life is a post-ethical plane of being. The ethical plane, as the Gītā dramatizes, is always a field of battle, with contending impulses and wants. Morality is significant to the extent that one finds multiplicity in the world. The enemy has to be engaged and overcome. But on the transcendental level, ethics loses its substance, once all empirical contradictions are transcended—cold and heat, pleasure and pain, praise and blame, and also, good and evil, right and wrong. This position is not antinomian. The person who has achieved the mystical state of *mokṣa* does not consciously follow the moral path, but neither can he or she deviate from it. Virtue is not victory through battle, it is the spontaneous overflow of wisdom. The Bhagavadgītā declares:

> The holy men whose sins are destroyed, whose doubts (dualities) are cut asunder, whose minds are disciplined and who rejoice in (doing) good to all creatures, attain to the beatitude of God.[19]

Thus love and compassion are the natural expression of enlightenment. This kind of knowledge helps one transcend mundane conflicts, but since through it one sees the divine in all things, it is no prescription for otherworldliness. To the contrary, social responsibilities are taken ever more seriously. Eminent philosophers, like Śaṁkara, have also been great humanitarians, not in spite of their philosophy but because of it.

In the remaining section we shall first highlight the cardinal principles of Hindu ethics, and then focus on its contextual orientation, which facilitates the task of making choices when dilemmas arise.

Cardinal Principles

The cardinal principles found in most Hindu sects are: purity, self-control, detachment, truth, and nonviolence. Each of these ideals has its own inner evolution and is therefore a mixture of ingredients not easily understandable to one unfamiliar with their cultural history. Thus, *purity* has a history of ritualism and ceremonialism, but progressively many of the rules pertaining to ablutions, food habits, and the like are internalized to signify the purity of mind and heart. So also, *self-control*, on one level, refers to the physical and mental senses. In the history of Hinduism such preoccupation has glorified asceticism and has made heroes of fanatics who have destroyed their sight glaring at the sun or atrophied their limbs through yogic acrobatics. On a higher level, self-control has gradually been perceived as a means for harmonizing all of one's calls and claims toward the development of a happy and healthy personality.

The ideal of *detachment* also has a long history, representing the perennial tension between the ideals of *dharma* and *mokṣa*—of world-affirmation and world-negation. The early Mīmāṁsā espoused the ideal of *dharma* so that the purpose of ethical action was that of enjoyment, both in this life and the next. The Mīmāṁsā consequently ridiculed ascetics who practiced renunciation. In time, under the influence of Jainism and Buddhism, Vedic orthodoxy adopted the *mokṣa* ideal and thereby ethics became the instrument for the attainment of liberation. However, even when it incorporated this new ideal into its philosophy, the Mīmāṁsā continued its former emphasis upon activity in the world. Against the objection that such activity, even when it is good, keeps one bound to the wheel of *saṁsāra* or rebirth, because a person must reap what is sown, the Mīmāṁsā responded that action performed in the spirit of detachment is emotionally empty and therefore not subject to the operation of karma.

The Bhagavad Gītā built on the ethical stance of the Mīmāṁsā. Its formulation of ethical activism is a refined synthesis of two orthodox though conflicting modes of discipline: *pravṛtti* (active life) and *nivṛtti* (quietism).

Devotees who embraced the first ideal engaged in Vedic rituals and duties prescribed by the Kalpa-sūtras with a view to reward in heaven. Devotees who embraced the second ideal abandoned all such works and relied solely on *jñaña* or knowledge as the pathway to liberation. They reasoned: since all actions—good or bad—must have their consequences in reincarnations, the most direct way to escape the pain of rebirth was to minimize all activity.

The Gītā counters the earlier argument that karma is evil and should be abandoned, because it leads to rebirth, by making a shrewd analysis of human behavior. It does not stop with karma, but goes beyond karma to *kāma*. Behind the deed lies the desire. Aversions and attachments determine a person's behavior, therefore an individual's real enemies are not actions but passions.[20] Actions are only the motor manifestations of the impulse to love or to hate.

The implication of this analysis is that the power to bind one to continued existence resides in *kāma*, not karma. Accordingly, karma without *kāma* has no consequence for rebirth. Once desire is removed from the deed, the deed loses its fateful sting. One who knows this is wise. He can work and yet do nothing that binds him. In the Gītā's words, "Having no desire, with his mind and self controlled, abandoning all possessions, performing actions with the body alone, he commits no sin."[21]

The Gītā's analysis of action as the extension of desire, along with the inference that detached action per se has no binding power, brings one to the conclusion that what is ethically required is not "renunciation of action" but "renunciation in action."[22]

The Gītā's nomenclature for detached activism is *karma-yoga*. *Karma-yoga* treats the act as an end in itself and not as a means to another end. The classic formulation of *karma-yoga* is embodied in the admonition, "In action only hast thou a right and never in its fruits. Let not thy motive be the fruits of action; nor let thy attachment be to inaction."[23]

Thus in the principle of *karma-yoga* the Gītā synthesizes the positive elements of *pravṛtti* and *nivṛtti*. "While it does not abandon activity, it preserves the spirit of renunciation. It commends the strenuous life, yet gives no room for the play of selfish impulses. Thus it discards neither ideal, but by combining them refines and ennobles both."[24]

The next two ideals, truth and nonviolence, are combined, and are regarded as Hinduism's highest ideals.

The ethical imperative of truthfulness flows from the metaphysical concept of Truth as Reality. Gandhi utters Upaniṣadic insight when he says, "Truth is by nature self-evident. As soon as you remove the cobwebs of ignorance that surround it, it shines clear."[25] Earlier, Gandhi believed that God is Truth, but subsequently he revised it to: Truth is God. By taking this step he felt he could include in the fold of believers all persons who were lovers of Truth and yet could not subscribe to any theistic ideology. His seeming innovation was not far removed from the Sanskrit word for Truth (*Sat*), which literally means "Being." The ontological meaning of *Sat* as "being" or "existing" is translated into the ethical meaning of *Sat* as "good."

The cardinal virtues reach their apex with the concept of *ahiṁsā*. It is *parama dharma* (highest virtue). The word is a compound of *a* = 'not' and *hiṁsā* = 'harmful.' It literally means, "Not to injure or harm." *Ahiṁsā* is a correlate of Hinduism's cosmic outlook and therefore its moral mandate comprehends the whole created order as being worthy of nonviolence.

As with the other cardinal virtues that have been tried and tested through the centuries, *ahiṁsā* has ancient origins. There is some speculation it began as a "protest against blood sacrifice." The ambitious Āryan settlers were hardly disposed to the values of *ahiṁsā*, judging by their records of wars and their aftermath. By the time of the Upaniṣads, when the meaning of sacrifice was ethicized, truthfulness and nonviolence were given prominence. The Chāndogya Upaniṣad says, "Austerity, almsgiving, uprightness, harmlessness, truthfulness—these are our gifts to the priests."[26] Strict adherence to *ahiṁsā* was observed by Buddhism, and more so by Jainism. Classical Hinduism, while maintaining the primacy of *ahiṁsā*, adjusted the ideal to social and political realities and developed a "just war" theory not unlike its Christian counterpart.

The strict interpretation of *ahiṁsā*, without qualifications or caveats, continued to appear in Hindu scriptural texts. For instance, in the the Yoga Sūtras of Patañjali, *ahiṁsā* provides the ethical framework for all the other virtues classified under *Yama* (restraint). *Ahiṁsā* is more than nonviolence, it is nonhatred (*vairatyagah*). Its scope is universal, and it cannot be relativized by a series of "ifs," "ands," or "buts."[27]

The individual, par excellence, who served as a bridge to bring the pristine character of *ahiṁsā* into the twentieth-century was Mahatama Gandhi (1869–1948). His innovation was the application of the principle of nonviolence to national and global affairs. *Satyagraha* (nonviolent protest) was the technique by which he took *ahiṁsā* out of the scriptures and on to the streets.

Gandhi acknowledged that "nonviolence is common to all religions," but found its highest expression and application in "Hinduism" which, for him, included Buddhism and Jainism. He declared, "Hinduism believes in the oneness not merely of all human life, but in the oneness of all that lives. Its worship of cow, is in my opinion, its unique contribution to the evolution of humanitarianism. It is a practical application of the belief in the oneness and, therefore, sacredness of all life."[28]

On the point of cow protection, Gandhi thought it was "the gift of Hinduism to the world." "It symbolized the protection of the weak by the strong. It subsumed everything that feels. Causing pain to the weakest creature on earth incurred a breach of the principle of cow protection."[29] Gandhi discovered nonviolence in his pursuit of Truth. He found that *ahiṁsā* and Truth were so intertwined that it was impossible to disentangle them. Even so, *ahiṁsā* was considered the means and Truth the end. "Means to be means must always be within our reach, and so ahiṁsā is our supreme duty. If we take care of the means, we are bound to reach the end sooner or later."[30]

This concludes our overview of Hindu ethics. Next we focus on certain distinctive features of Hindu ethics that uniquely equip it in the task of doing bioethics.

Contextual Structure of Hindu Ethics

Any survey of clinical cases reveals that dilemmas lie at the heart of bioethics. For its part, Hindu ethics is a moral system that acknowledges genuine moral dilemmas. We encounter a dilemma when values to which we are equally committed are brought into conflict, so that the honoring of one value necessitates the violation of the other. Western ethicists admit that moral dilemmas are the Achilles heel of most problems encountered in bioethics. Beauchamp cites the classic case of Socrates in prison, sentenced to die. His friend Crito offers him an escape route with many good reasons to justify his act of breaking the law. Socrates countered with equally weighty reasons to support his own position to respect law and stay. The illustration serves to highlight the central problem of bioethics. "The reasons on each side are weighty ones, and neither is in any obvious way the right set of reasons. If we act on either set of reasons, our actions will be desirable in some respects but undesirable in other respects. And yet we think that ideally we ought to act on all of these reasons, for each is, considered by itself, a good reason."[31]

The Hindu position is to be distinguished both from the *religious fundamentalist*, who views dilemmas in the light of revelation, and the *secular rationalist*, who views them as problems to be solved by the use of reason. For the religious fundamentalist, the problem is the need for better faith; for the secular rationalist, it is the need for superior knowledge. In either case, there are no genuine dilemmas.

In Hinduism, dilemmas are not denied. Its scriptures strain with the tension of irreconcilable alternatives. The best examples are found in the epic literature. The Mahābhārata and the Rāmāyaṇa are not just works of antiquity but embody the social sinew that connects past with present and makes the epics dateless treasuries of true dilemmas.

The Bhagavad Gītā opens with a moral dilemma tugging at the heart and mind of Arjuna, as this lonesome warrior faces the choice of having to kill or be killed by his own kinsmen. Bimal K. Matilal in his *Moral Dilemmas in the Mahabharata* transports us to another episode in the life of Arjuna in which he confronts the difficult claims of promise keeping versus fratricide.

> On the very day of final encounter between Karṇa and Arjuna Yudhiṣṭhira fled the battelfield after being painfully humiliated by Karna in an armed engagement. When Arjuna came to the camp to pay visit to him and asked what really happened, Yudhiṣṭhira flared up in anger and told Arjuna that all his boastfulness about being the finest archer in the world was a lot of nonsense because the war was dragging on. He reminded Arjuna that the latter claimed to be capable of conquering everybody and thus end the war within a few days. In a rage, he not only insulted Arjuna but also slighted the "Gāṇḍiva bow," the most precious possession of this valiant warrior. The bow was a gift to Arjuna from Agni, the fire-god. He held it so dear to his heart that he had promised to kill anyone whou would ever speak ill of "Gāṇḍiva."[32]

Yudhiṣṭhira's vehemence put Arjuna in a tight corner where he would either have to kill his elder brother or break his promise. "When his Kṣatriya duty (dharma) made him choose the first alternative, Kṛṣṇa (his alter ego) appeared. On being asked, Arjuna explained: he was obliged to commit fratricide in order to fulfil his obligation to keep his promise."[33] His strong sense of duty made Arjuna reduce the situation to a moral conflict in which duty must prevail. To be sure, the duty of promise keeping was inviolable—the moral equivalent of protecting the truth (*satyarakṣā*). Matilal observes that the scenario resonates with Kantian ethics, which also gives highest priority to truth telling.[34] But Kṛṣṇa was no Kant. He argued with Arjuna that "promise-keeping or even truth-telling cannot be an unconditional obligation when it is in conflict with the avoidance of grossly unjust and criminal acts such as patricide or fratricide. Saving an innocent life is also a strong obligation; saving his elder brother would naturally be an equally strong obligation, if not stronger. Hence, in fact, according to Kṛṣṇa, two almost equally strong obligations or duties are in conflict here."[35]

In all such conflicts, the *dharmic* thing to do is to be guided by the *demands of the situation*. There is no question about the need to maintain the consistency of an ethical system, but sometimes the infraction of these virtues is permitted to achieve noble ends. This does not reduce ethics to opportunism; but neither is it made the hostage of absolutism.

The point is illustrated by Kṛṣṇa's story about Kauśika, a hermit who had taken a vow always to speak the truth. One day, while seated at a crossroad, this holy man was begged by a band of fleeing travelers not to divulge their escape route to bandits in hot pursuit, with intentions to take their lives. Kauśika did not reply. When the bandits arrived at the scene, knowing fully well that the hermit could not tell a lie, they asked about the travelers, and Kauśika told them the truth. The travelers were caught and killed. Kauśika's fate was equally sad. Though he had punctiliously practiced virtue in order to reach heaven, he failed to achieve his goal, because, in this instance, truthtelling was a violent act that emptied his store of merit. Clearly the demand of the situation was the overriding duty to save precious lives, even though to effect this meant recourse to dissimulation. But Kauśika was an absolutist who could not see that truth telling ceased being an unconditional obligation when weighed in the balance with the need for preserving lives.[36]

The Mahābhārata recounts numerous other instances illustrating the relativity of moral conduct in the context of "duties in distress." A Brāhmaṇa in distress is allowed to perform sacrifice even for an unworthy person, and may eat prohibited food. A Kṣatriya, unable to subsist by his caste duties when his own avocation is destroyed, is allowed to engage in the duties of a Vaiśya, taking to agriculture and cattle rearing. The Śantiparvan declares it is not sinful to drink alchohol for medical purposes, to accede to a preceptor's wish to cohabit with his wife for the purpose of raising progeny, to steal in a time of emergency, to tell lies to robbers, and so on.[37]

Similar exceptions are permitted by Manu, the greatest exponent of orthodox morality. Personal survival is deemed higher than the stealing of property, making it justifiable for a hungry person to steal food when all other measures fail.[38] Following Manu, other Dharmaśāstra writers permit perjury to save life as an act of dharma.

However, notwithstanding the dharmic justification of lying and other such acts in situations of moral conflict, Hindu ethics strictly enjoins the maintenance of its integrity in keeping with the *puruṣārthas* or values of life. These values are integrated and progressive, culminating in the *summum bonum* of liberation.

Thus the internal flexibility of Hindu ethics gives it a certain advantage over two extreme positions on the current social spectrum, dealing with life-and-death issues.

First there is the position of *authoritarianism*. It surfaces in different degrees in the moral stance of religious groups such as the Roman Catholic Chuch, Protestant fundamentalists, Mormons, and Operation Rescue, an activist organization responsible for the bombing of several birth control clinics. These groups base their truth claims on holy books in which they find objectively valid norms of conduct. They see human reason as flawed, and therefore rely on revelation for the truth, the whole truth, and nothing but the truth. This makes them tend to see moral issues in terms of black and white, and therefore to have little tolerance for exceptional cases.

At the opposite end of the spectrum is the position of *relativism*. Relativists argue that value judgments and ethical norms are reducible to matters of subjective preference, and therefore questions of life and death are considered private issues to be answered by each individual. They, too, minimize the capacity of reason. With hedonic overtones, relativists make the individual's own experience of happiness the standard of value, worthy of protection by the American Constitution.

Hindu ethics is distinguished from both extremes by the importance it gives to *rational authority*. This claim may be queried because of the part played by revelation within its own system. However, Hinduism's recognition of revelation as a conduit of knowledge does not depreciate the role of reason. The Hindu *śāstras* make a liberal use of reason in support of the positions they take. Only the final validity of reason is questioned in mystical matters that lie beyond its purview. Thus the admission of revelation does not prejudice reason, for there is continuity between the two. Whereas in Western thought revelation is an external mode of testimony, in Hindu perspective revelation is an internal activity, similar to intuition. "It begins, no doubt, as an external opinion inasmuch as we appropriate it from a guru. But we do not merely acquiesce in it. We are under an obligation to intuit it and make it our own, when it will cease to be external and become inwardly as clear to us as it is to our teacher."[39]

Through reason and intuition, Hinduism finds the source of ethics in the *nature of the person, holistically perceived*. It agrees with the relativists that the claims of authoritarianism to finding absolute values are illusory and pretentious, because social morality is inevitably the construct of subjective, historical forces that reflect the accidents of time and place; but this admission of subjectivity is not tantamount to saying that all of our choices between life and death are merely the products of subjective preferences. To the contrary, we can arrive at objectively valid norms based on our knowledge of deep-seated human capacties for life, for love, for freedom, and for integrity. Our cultural formulations of these psychic strivings will always be relative, constantly to be refined over the long haul of human experience—which is to acknowledge that objectivity is not absolute or unconditional. The notion of *absolutism is alien to Hindu ethics*, because it is a concept of transcendental revelation that is removed from an appreciative understanding of human nature and human history.

This approach imparts to Hindu bioethics a *contextual orientation of moral reasoning* in its dealings with moral problems. It eschews the paths of authoritarianism, creedalism, emotionalism, and takes the road of rationality. However it is not the rationality of the disembodied mind, but the rationality of the whole person. The autonomous individual gives due weight to scriptural injunctions and the precedents of persons of probity, but in the final analysis he turns to his own conscience, guided by what collective religious experience has defined as being of ultimate value.

Notwithstanding its claim to rationality, Hindu bioethics acknowledges that persons of reason might not always agree on what is good, but they can agree more generally on what is evil. Rational people wish to avoid for themselves and for their loved ones evils such as pain, disease, premature death, and the loss of abilities to do what one wants to do. Therefore, while promoting the good, the basic agenda of Hindu bioethics is to prevent evil by advocating principles and proscriptions against behavior that inflicts harm to persons and all sentient creatures. Its bottom line is: Do no harm—*hiṃsaṃ mā kuru.*

The vehicle that brings Hindu ethics into the new world of bioethics is the notion of *dharma*. This we have seen is not some static moral concept, standing palely for the values of India in a bygone time with little relevance for other peoples and other places. *Dharma* is a catalyst for change. It preserves order in the midst of change, and change in the midst of order; and thereby is always on the side of progress. For further discussion of ideas presented here the reader is referred to my *Dilemmas of Life and Death* (see Bibliography) in which the arguments of the concluding section appear.

Fuller treatments of Hindu ethics may be found in my earlier works on which portions of the Introduction depends: *The Evolution of Hindu Ethical Ideals* (Hawaii: The University Press of Hawaii, 1982), *In Search of Hinduism* (UTS Press, 1986) *World Religions and Global Ethics* (New York: Paragon House, 1989), and *Dilemmas of Life and Death, Hindu Ethics in a North American Context* (New York: State University of New Press, 1995).

CHAPTER 2

INDIAN MEDICINE

ANCIENT INDIAN MEDICAL LORE

A unique feature of Hinduism is that a fully fledged system of medicine evolved within its complex ethos. The historical developments are shrouded in mystery due to their long antiquity. Yet, inasmuch as all primitive societies have survived by recourse to some rudimentary system of medicine, it is fair to assume that during the protohistoric Harappa Culture, which preceded and followed 2000 B.C., a rudimentary system of medicine was practiced in the northwestern region of India. Archaeological excavations at the two main capitals of Harappa and Mohenjodaro give evidence of a technically advanced society that built its houses, streets, and public facilities with a knowledge of the principles of good hygiene and sanitation. Water was valued for its purifying and therapeutic qualities. Terra cotta figurines and images on seals suggest powerful sentiments for Mother Earth and her bounty of plants and animals. The figure of a horned deity, ritualistically seated in a yogic position, typifies an ancient medicine-man, and is thought to be the forerunner of Śiva, a later Hindu god who is worshipped as Lord of Beasts (*Pāsúpati*). The written records of this period have not yet been deciphered, which makes it impossible to arrive at any actual knowledge of its medical lore, but it may be suggested that, "as in many other features of Indian life, the Harappa Culture contained the seeds of much that was characteristic of later Indian medicine."[1]

The Harappa Culture collapsed by around 1500 B.C.E., probably due to the invasions of Āryan tribes from the north. Data covering the end of the second millenium B.C.E. are drawn from the Ṛg Veda, the earliest literature of India, which gives us clearer glimpses of the state of medicine in the early Vedic period.

Intimations of medical lore in the Ṛg Veda are found in various myths that narrate the healing prowess of the vedic deities: Aśvins, Rudra, Soma, and Varuṇa. The last mentioned god is preeminently of moral character. Varuṇa is a gracious healer, but he also punishes with disease the violators of moral law. Thus a link is early formed between behavior ("sin") and disease conceived as the punitive visitation of the gods. More generally, all morbid states of body and mind that could not be attributed to divine agency or to circumstances were assigned to demonic forces. Other causes of disease were the breach of taboos or the result of sorcery and witchcraft. In addition to these theories of the origin of disease through external agencies, benevolent or malevolent, there is a more rational explanation of morbidity in terms of worms and insects that occupy the organism. Allowances were made for wounds and fractures incurred by accident or in war.

The diagnosis of disease involved a careful tabulation of repetitive symptoms that helped identify the offending demon, who was then removed through healing rituals. Amulets of plants or herbs were worn to prevent the demon from reentry. Vedic belief in the curative efficacy of herbs and plants made for the development of an elaborate pharmacopeia. Since the healing rituals were conducted in correlation with the movement of stars and planets, it is assumed that astrology also played a part in Vedic medicine.

The medical professional during the latter part of the second millenium B.C. was the *bhiṣaj*, whose name was later identified with the *vaidya*—a title that is still used today. It is possible that the *bhiṣaj* was originally a bone-setter, as Filliozat contends,[2] but that role was soon expanded, because references to his use of healing herbs suggest that his practice took on other specialties.[3] His special knowledge was rewarded with payments of horses, cattle, and domestic amenities.

More important than the Ṛg Veda for knowledge of ancient Indian medical lore are the hymns of the Atharva Veda, which should be read with the Kauśikasūtra. In these hymns the diseases and also their remedies are invoked as supernatural beings. Through spells and incantations the worshipper attempts to avoid harm or secure blessings. In addition to charms and spells, herbs are used as curative agents. Skillful use of homeopathic and allopathic principles are employed in healing.

Vedic medicine was predominantly magico-religious, but mixed in with sorcery and witchcraft are certain empirical facets of healing. These procedures include surgery; methods for stopping hemorrhage; bonesetting; hydrotherapy; and extensive use of plants and herbs. Underlying a good deal of the ritualistic actions is a clever use of the power of suggestion and of visualization.[4]

During the millenium preceding the Christian era, developments took place that precipitated a paradigm shift from the earlier magico-religious tradition to the new empirico-rational medicine of Āyurveda. Here we must point out that sharp differences of opinion exist among scholars. On the one hand there are representatives of traditional Indian medicine who hold the view that Indian medicine was a brahmanic science from the very beginning. This view is now challenged by Indologists such as the eminent writer in Āyurvedic studies, Kenneth G. Zysk. In his groundbreaking text, *Asceticism and Healing in Ancient India* (1991), Zysk sets out to investigate the crucial period from 800 to 100 B.C.E.[5] The book attempts to understand "the socioreligious dynamics during this period, which saw the transition from Vedic medicine, anchored in magico-religious ideology, to Āyurveda, dominated by an empirico-rational epistemology." The methodology of the book involves a historical and philological exploration of diverse Indian and non-Indian sources, especially Buddhist materials. By critically examining these sources, Zysk concludes that the traditional position of teachers and authors of Āyurveda who claim that it was a brahmanic science from its inception "results from Hindu intellectual endeavors to render a fundamentally heterodox science orthodox."[6] Zysk points out that in early Vedic beginnings "medicine and healers were excluded from the core of the orthodox brahmanic social and religious hierarchy and found acceptance among the heterodox traditions of mendicant ascetics, or *śramaṇas*, who became the repository of a vast storehouse of medical knowledge."[7] Feeling no need to bow to brahmanic prohibitions and taboos, "these sramanic physicians developed an empirically based medical epistemology and accumulated medical lore from different healing traditions in ancient India."[8]

Zysk traces the contribution made by Buddhism to Indian medicine through its institutionalization in monasteries, which led to new models for medical manuals; through the emergence of monk-healers; and through the establishment of monastic hospices and infirmaries. All of these factors aided the popularization of Buddhism throughout the subcontinent during the reign of Asóka.

Zysk concludes: "Hinduism assimilated the ascetic medical repository into its socioreligious and intellectual tradition beginning probably during the Gupta period and by the application of a brahmanic veneer made it an orthodox Hindu science."[9]

The argument presented here is for the most part valid. There is ample evidence that Buddhist and Jain scholars aided in the development of medical science, inasmuch as their anti-brahmanical philosophy afforded them the freedom and impetus to experiment without risk of breaking taboos. However, Zysk tends to overlook and underestimate the interactive capacity of Hindu ideas and ideals, and their ability to adapt to new findings, especially in the medical field. The naturalistic orientation of Hindu medicine, given its philosophic underpinnings, probably made it easier to assimilate heterodox views in ways not possible for more traditional branches of Hinduism.

ĀYURVEDA

Definition

Āyurveda is "the science of (living to a ripe) age." The term is semantically significant. Basham notes: "Its first component (*āyur*) implies that the ancient Indian doctor was concerned not only with curing disease but also with promoting positive health and longevity, while the second (*veda*) has religious overtones, being the term used for the most sacred texts of Hinduism."[10] It is specifically associated with the Atharva Veda (CS Su.11.6).

Tradition

Like the legends that describe the origins of other Indian sciences, Āyurveda is molded in myth. Filliozat remarks: "Almost upto our times, it has been an Indian practice to take back the first teaching of sciences and letters to superior gods."[11] And so the script becomes an invention of Brahman, astrology is ascribed to Sūrya, the grammar of Pāṇini was elaborated by Śiva, and learning comes from Indra.

In the case of Āyurveda, Caraka traces its dissemination to the outbreak of diseases, which impeded all aspects of human activites and limited the lifespan of living beings. The crisis captured the sympathy of sages who "assembled on one of the auspicious sides of the Himalayas" to hold deliberations. There was consensus that "disease-free condition is the best source of virtue, wealth, gratification and emancipation, while diseases are destroyers of this [source], welfare and life itself."[12] The sages then delegated Bharadvāja to enlist the help of god Indra, who had received medical knowledge from the Ashvins, heavenly physicians, and who in turn had been instructed by the Creator (Brahmā) himself.

Lord Indra delivered to Bharadvāja the core of Āyurveda, containing knowledge pertaining to etiology, symptomatology, and therapeutics of both the healthy and unhealthy states of a person. Bharadvāja passed the science on to Ātreya Punarvasu and other seers. Ātreya trained six disciples in the science, including Agniveśa, who preserved the doctrine of Ātreya in the Agniveśa Tantra. This composition was reconstructed by Caraka. Sections of Caraka's revision were either not finished or lost. Dṛḍhabala made his own revisions (approximately A.D. 500), finishing the last two of eight books and seventeen chapters of the sixth book.[13]

The myth of the apocalypse of Āyurveda, preserved in popular memory and buried deep in the Hindu psyche, offers many insights. We highlight a few:

- All living organisms are regulated by the principles of pleasure and pain.
- The yearnings for permanent happiness and freedom from pain, or, at least, the avoidance and alleviation of suffering, are universal and eternal.
- All living beings have been created for health.
- Disease is an impediment to the fulfillment of all human goals, including the spiritual.
- The quest for longevity is a moral obligation we owe to ourselves and to other persons with whom we are connected in the human family.[14]
- The gods function as paradigms, exemplifying through their empathy how humans should act—"*Iti deva akurvata ity u vau manusyah.*"
- The ultimate goal of medicine is the relief of human suffering.
- Sickness and death should serve as constant reminders of our common bonds and need for one another.

Divisions

Caraka states that Āyurveda was divided into eight branches:

1. Internal medicine *(Kāyacikitsā)*
2. Surgery *(Śalyāpahartṛka)*
3. Diseases of the supraclavicular area *(Śalakya)*

4. Pediatrics—including obstetrics/gynecology *(Kaumārabhṛtya)*
5. Toxicology *(Viṣagaravairodhikapraśamana)*
6. Psychiatry *(Bhūtavidyā)*
7. Rejuvenation *(Rasāyana)*
8. Knowledge for increase of virility *(Vājīkaraṇa)*[15]

As each branch developed, it became a specialized discipline, but an interdisciplinary approach ensured that each part was reckoned as belonging to the whole. Two disciplines developed in time into fully fledged schools: *Kāyacikitsā* or the School of Medicine and *Śalyā* or the School of Surgery.

Sources

The most authoritative texts on Āyurveda are certain extant collections known as the Great Trio (*Bṛhat-Trayī*). They are (1) the *Caraka Saṃhitā* (2) the *Suśruta Saṃhitā*, and (3) Vāgbhaṭa's *Aṣṭāngahṛdayam.* Note: our primary sources, listed in full in the Bibliography, include *Caraka-Saṃhitā* (3 vols.), Priyavarat Sharma, editor-translator; *The Suśruta Saṃhitā* (3 vols.), Kaviraj Kunjalal Bhishagratna, editor-translator; *Aṣṭānga Hṛdayam* (2 vols.). Secondary sources, on which we have relied for translation of terms and medical descriptions, include *Caraka Saṃhitā: A Scientific Synopsis*, P. Ray, H. N. Gupta, editors, and *Suśruta Saṃhitā*: A Scientific Synopsis, P. Ray, H. N.Gupta, M. Roy, editors.

The Caraka Saṃhitā

The Caraka Saṃhitā (treatise compiled by Caraka) is a Sanskrit work of great antiquity. The original composition has undergone two redactions at different times, which makes it difficult to fix an accurate date. Winternitz sets it at 100 A.D., and that is followed by the Chronology Committee of the National Institute of Sciences of India.[16]

The contents of the treatise cover an elaborate diversity of diseases, along with their etiology, diagnosis, prognosis, and treatment. It discusses several theoretical and practical areas of medicine, including embryology, obstetrics, anatomy, physiology, personal hygiene, sanitation, and the training and duties of physicians. It claims to know all that is to be known of therapeutic medicine. Its main focus is on Āyurveda, but integrated with the science of life is an exposition of philosophic concepts that provide the fundamental assumptions behind the knowledge and practice of medicine in ancient India.

The scope of the Caraka Saṃhitā covers ten specific subjects. They are:

1. Anatomy *(Śarīra)*
2. Physiology *(Vṛtti)*
3. Etiology *(Hetu)*
4. Pathology *(Vyādhi)*
5. Treatment *(Karma)*
6. Objectives *(Kārya)*
7. Impact of age and season *(Kāla)*
8. Physicians *(Kartri)*
9. Medicine and instruments *(Karaṇa)*
10. Procedure and sequence *(Vidhiviniścaya)*[17]

The saṃhitā is divided into eight sections to facilitate discussion of the above subjects:

- *Sūtrasthānam* (on fundamentals): drugs, health, precepts, preparations, diseases, food/drink.
- *Nidānasthānam* (diagnosis): of fevers, hemorrhage, urine disorders, phthisis, epilepsy.
- *Vimānasthānam* (specific features): of rasā, epidemics, of diseases, of therapeutics.
- *Śārīrasthānam* (anatomy and embryology): types of persons, descent of embryo, fetal development, procreation.
- *Indriyasthānam* (signs of life and death): complexion and voice, smell, taste, palpation, shadow and luster, conditions of eyes, nose, teeth.
- *Cikitsāsthānam* (therapeutics): rasāyana, aphrodisiacs, fevers, internal hemorrhage, abdominal lumps, skin disorders, insanity, wounds, swellings, anemia, diarrhea, vomiting, erysipelas, poisoning, alchoholism, disorders of female genitals, defects of semen.
- *Kalpasthānam* (pharmacy) pharmaceutical preparations.
- *Siddhisthānam* (cure of diseases): sussessful preparation, pancakarma, enemas, emesis, purgation, post-enematic conditions.[18]

There is a total of one hundred and fifty chapters dealing with specific subjects.

Suśruta Saṃhitā

The Suśruta Saṃhitā is distinguished as being the earliest known treatise dealing extensively with surgery, an area that is treated lightly by Caraka.

Its excellence lies in its rational and systematic approach to the many subjects covered in the field. Its origins are obscure; the extant work is a recension by the alchemist Nāgārjuna from an earlier text. The date of the recension by Nāgārjuna has been set as being from the third to fourth centuries A.D. by the Chronology Committee of the National Institute of Sciences of India.[19]

The Suśruta Saṃhitā affirms the purpose of Āyurveda as combining the cure of disease with the preservation of health to ensure a long, happy, and useful life. It incorporates the eight branches of Āyurveda we have listed earlier, but accords surgery special importance as being the most ancient branch of medicine and capable of producing immediate results.[20]

The Suśruta Saṃhitā has one hundred and twenty chapters in five divisions. They are:

- *Sūtrasthāna* (fundamental postulates)
- *Nidānasthāna* (pathology)
- *Sārīrasthāna* (embryology and anatomy)
- *Cikitsāsthāna* (medical treatment)
- *Kalpasthāna* (toxicology)
- The concluding sections, *Uttaratantra* (specialized knowledge) are the contribution of the redactor Nāgārjuna to the original text.[21]

Indian surgery owes a dubious debt to Vedic sacrifices, which supplied good knowledge of comparative anatomy. Suśruta's skills in practical surgery were based on his knowledge of practical anatomy. He classified his operations into five categories: extractions of solid bodies; excising; incising; probing; scarifying; suturing; puncturing; and removing fluids. These surgeries were performed with the use of some one hundred and twenty-five instruments.[22]

Suśruta specialized in plastic and rhinoplastic operations; lithotomic operations; amputations; ophthalmic surgery; midwifery; and dissection.

Given the holistic orientation of Indian medicine, it is not surprising to find Suśruta also discussing such questions as the nature and destiny of human life, and man's place in the universe.

The Aṣṭānga Hṛdayam

The Aṣṭāngahṛdaya of Vāgbhaṭa (quintessence of the eight branches of Āyurveda) is the last of the triad of authoritative texts on ancient Indian medicince. Its translator says: "With its beauty and brevity of poetical composition, sequential arrangement of topics, clear description of precepts and practices of medical science and many other merits, it has earned its rightful place as one among the *Bṛhat trayī* (three great treatises) of Āyurveda."[23] Its popularity, as a summary of Āyurveda, lies in the fact that it has a higher number of commentaries than any other Āyurvedic treatise. Vāgbhaṭa was a Buddhist (perhaps a later convert from Hinduism), who belonged to the middle of the seventh century.

The Aṣṭāṅgahṛdaya has six sections, comprising one hundred and twenty chapters, and is composed entirely in poetry. The six sections are:

1. *Sūtrasthāna*: basic doctrines; principles of health, prevention of diseases; diet; drugs; physiology; pathology; diseases and their treatment.
2. *Śārirasthāna*: embryology; anatomy; physiology; physical and psychological constitutions; inauspicious dreams and omens; signs of oncoming death.
3. *Nidānasthāna*: causes of disease; premonitory symptoms; characteristic features of diseases; pathogenesis and prognosis of disease.
4. *Cikitsāsthāna*: treatment of diseases; medicinal recipes; diet; care of patients.
5. *Kalpasiddhisthāna*: preparation of recipes; purificactory therapies; management of complications; principles of pharmacy.
6. *Uttarasthāna*: pediatrics; psychiatry; diseases of the head; opthalmology; surgery; toxicology; rejuvenation therapy; virilification therapy.[24]

In 1890 a medical manuscript in fourth-century characters was discovered in Turkestan, known as the Bower Manuscript. It offers proof that Āyurveda was fully established as a science by that time.[25] By the ninth century, the texts of Caraka, Suśruta, and Vāgbhaṭa were carried beyond India and were known to Arabic medical circles. Evidence for this comes from citations in the *Firdaus al-Hikmat* by Abul Hasan Ali bin Rabbani Tabari, compiled in A.D. 856. Thus "Indian medicine reached its classical form in the early centuries of the Christian era, the period crowned by the dynasty of the imperial Guptas, when the level of Indian culture was at its highest."[26]

The Ethical Orientation of Indian Medicine

Our brief introduction to the medical manuals of Āyurveda impress us for the range of topics they cover, reading almost like modern medical texts, notwithstanding their antiquity; and also for their concern for the moral dimensions of medicine. This orientation bodes well for our attempt to construct a system of Hindu bioethics.

This symbiosis between medicine and morals follows from common philosophical assumptions that underlie both disciplines. Before we introduce the Indian medical system, we highlight some of its salient features that provide the bases for ethical analysis:

- Āyurveda is rational in its approach to medicine. In place of the supernatural therapy (*daiva-vyapāśraya*) of the Vedic phase, it introduced rational therapy (*yukti-vyapāśraya*) to make the system logical and scientific.
- Āyurveda is holistic. It views the person as an integrated whole and not just an aggregate of several body parts that are the domain of specialists.
- Āyurveda sees the person as grounded in nature: a microcosm within the macrocosm. Diet, climate, soil, season, time, and place are all factors with which to reckon.
- Health and healing are regarded as acts of nature. In medico-ethical terms: the natural is the good.
- Health is identified as a positive state, and not just the absence of disease.
- Health is multidimensional: physical, mental, social, and spiritual.
- Āyurveda apprehends the person as an individual, having a unique constitutional type, and as the bearer of an unmatched set of life experiences.
- Āyurveda gives prominence to the notion of balance. It promotes an ethics of moderation in matters of sex and abstinence, food and drink, work and play, sleeping and awaking, faith and common sense.
- Medicine is essentialy preventive and promotive, elevating caring above curing.
- Longevity is measured not in numbers of days, but quality of time.
- Death is an inevitable part of the natural process, and is therefore not an evil or the object of divine punishment. Death is the opposite of birth, not of life.
- Health and disease, happiness and suffering, life and death are the consequences of an individual's karma, hence the emphasis on human responsibility.

- Health is more than what the doctor does; it is a total life-style that carries one from cradle to the grave.[27]
- Health is not the ultimate good but the penultimate good.

The moral structure of Indian medicine makes it eminently suited to deal with the dilemmas that arise in modern medical practice. Next we turn to the conceptual and theoretical framework in which these ideas are set.

Basic Concepts and Theories of Āyurveda

Aim of Medical Science

The entire medical enterprise of Āyurveda is governed by a philosophic understanding of the person. The individual is conceived as "an epitome of the macrocosm." Both the microcosm and macrocosm are manifestations of Brahman. Spirit and matter are not dichotomized, but belong to "one integral whole." They share a common constitution of six elements: earth, water, fire, air, and ether. The sixth element, which represents the spirit or self in the individual is equal to Brahman in the universe (Sa.5.5). "Similar to the office of the creator in the universe is the might of the individual soul in man. He also creates life by the act of impregnation (Sa.5.6). Like the diverse things present in the universe, the different entities comprising the human being are too numerous to count (Sa.5.6). There is in man as much diversity as in the world outside (Sa. 5.3)."[28]

To gain the knowledge of Brahman and thereby to achieve spiritual freedom, the individual cannot rely on rituals and ascetical practices of conventional religion, but must build a sound mind in a sound body. It is this soteriological context that gives medicine its mandate.

In the process, the aim of Āyurveda is to supply accurate information pertaining to what makes a life happy (*sukha-āyus*) and beneficial (*hita-āyus*) and what makes it unhappy (*dukkha-āyus*) and harmful (*ahita-āyus*). Āyurveda presents data on factors that produce these four types of life and on what enhances the life span.[29]

In his definition of *āyus*, Caraka states:

> Life is said as happy if the person is not afflicted with any somatic or psychic disorder, is particularly youthful, capable with energy, reputation, manliness and prowess, possessing knowledge, specific knowledge and strong organs and sense objects; having immense wealth and various favourable enjoyments, has achieved desired results of all actions and moves about where he likes. Contrary to it is unhappy life.

> Life is said as beneficial if the person is well-wisher of all the creatures, abstains from taking other's possession, is truth-speaking, calm, taking steps after examining the situation, free from carelessness, observing the three categories (virtue, wealth and enjoyment) without their mutual conflict, worshiping the worthy persons, is devoted to knowledge, understanding and serenity of mind, keeping company of the elderly persons, has controlled well the impulses of attachment, aversion, envy, intoxication and conceit, is engaged in various types of gifts, constantly devoted to penance, knowledge and peace, has knowledge of and devotion to metaphysics, keeping eye to both the worlds and is endowed with memory and intelligence. Contrary to it is non-beneficial life.[30]

Commenting on this formulation of the aims of Āyurveda, P. V. Sharma highlights its social dimension: "It is clear that a person should be healthy and happy personally but, at the same time, he should also be useful for the society, otherwise his life cannot be taken as meaningful. From this it is quite evident that Āyurveda is conscious not only to personal health of the individual but also to social medicine which is concerned with the health of the community."[31]

In summary, human life is multidimensional, and is lived, simultaneously, on different levels. On the material level, Āyurveda is involved with the maintenance of a healthy state of balance of all elements of the human organism and their restoration when they become deranged. On the psychic level, it cultivates a rational approach to life, removing ignorance that brings harm, and supplying information that keeps one happy and useful to a ripe, old age. On the spiritual level, Āyurveda provides healthful conditions of mind and body for the progressive achievement of all of one's capacities, until the human mind realizes its identity with Ultimate Reality. In fine: "Āyurveda attempts a co-ordinated and harmonized three-fold pursuit of happy material existence, proper secular conduct, and spiritual salvation through a correct understanding of the true relationship between man, his world, and the ultimate source of his consciousness and existence."[32]

Philosophy and Psychology

Āyurveda is a compendium of science and philosophy. As a science its purpose is to ensure health of body and mind, but as a philosophy its goals go beyond the preservation of health and the curing of disease. The present resurgence of Āyurveda in the West is as much due to its philosophy as its science, because it appeals to the felt need for a more humanistically oriented approach to medicine.

Dasgupta raises the issue as to whether the speculations in the medical schools deserve to be included in a history of Indian philosophy. In his judgment any objection loses its force when it is remembered that "medicine was the most important of all the physical sciences which were cultivated in ancient India, was directly and intimately connected with the Sāṁkhya and Vaiśeṣika physics and was probably the origin of the logical speculations subsequently codified in the Nyāya-sūtras."[33] He proceeds to point out that the medical literature embodies a vision of life that is supported by interesting ethical instructions not present in works on philosophy. The manuals also cover many other interesting details that "throw a flood of lights on the scholastic methods of Indian thinkers." Moreover, scholars in touch with "the importance of Hatha Yoga or Tantra physiology or anatomy in relation to some of the Yoga practices of those schools will no doubt be interested to know for purposes of comparison or contrast the speculations of the medical schools on kindred points of interest." Dasgupta concludes his case for the inclusion of the medical literature in his *History of Indian Philosophy* by arguing that even "a student of pure philosophy" will find intriguing the medical speculations regarding "embryology, heredity and other such points of general enquiry."[34]

Dasgupta's remarks highlight the fact that the development of medicine in India has gone hand in hand with the development of philosophy. The reason for this is that Indian philosophy is more than intellectual curiosity; it is the quest for the elimination of moral and physical suffering that characterizes all of human existence. The goal of philosophy is to liberate the human consciousness to its native level of being; and sound health, as we have seen, is the sine qua non of this philosophic end. This inclusion of knowledge and wisdom, with paths to attain liberation, has distinguished Indian philosophy as "a way of life and not merely a way of thought." K. N. Udupa reminds us that the most characteristic path prescribed for reaching *mokṣa* has been a cultivation of the spirit of renunciation. The progressive practice of renunciation internally produces peace of mind and externally transforms behavior. This gradually produces empathy for all of life, in keeping with the principle of *ahiṁsā,* which is integral to the Hindu faith. Such a faith is not only directed toward the welfare of human beings, but also toward all living creatures whom human beings are obligated to serve, by virtue of their position of privilege.[35]

Āyurveda draws primarily from the philosophies of Sāṁkhya and Vaiśeṣika, but also in lesser degree from Vedānta, Nyāya, Yoga, Jain, and

Buddhist systems. As to the extent and nature of these borrowings, Larson states, "It is not the case that the ancient Indian medical theorizing represents a 'tight' or 'hard' appropriation of these classical *darśana-s*. Medical practitioners undoubtedly knew their philosophies, and it is clear enough from the use of terminology that they understood the classical *darśana*-s in technical detail. It is also clear, however, they utilized the technicalities of Indian philosophy for their own purposes even if that meant stretching various conceptualizations beyond the parameters of precise philosophical usage."[36]

Taking a cue from the Vaiśeṣika philosophy, Caraka states, "*Āyus* means the conjunction of body, sense organs, mind and self and is known by the synonyms *dhari*, *jivita, nityaga and anubandha*."[37] Thus *Āyus* (life) is not a simple form of being, but the integration of several components.

The body *(śarīra)* is constituted of four atomic substances *(bhūta):* earth *(pṛthvī),* water *(ap),* fire *(tejas),* and wind *(vāyu);* and three all-pervasive substances: space *(ākāśa),* time *(kāla),* and extension *(dis).*

The mind *(manas, sattva)* is localised in the body. It is also an atomic substance, inasmuch as its attention is finite and limited, and it has the ability to move, as in transmigration.

The self *(ātman),* by contrast, is all-pervasive. When it comes into relationship with the atomic mind, it produces consciousness *(cetanā),* and makes possible the operation of karma.

Together, the body, mind, and self form a tripod *(trindandavat).* Out of this threefold association *(samyoga),* life *(āyus)* arises. This is *puruṣa,* the person, which is the whole object of Āyurveda. The Kaṭha Upaniṣad describes this association through the simile of the chariot.[38]

In the Parable of the Chariot *(Ratha-rūpaka),* the soul *(ātman)* is the owner of the chariot, which is the body. The driver is *buddhi* (reason, intellect), *or vijñāna* (discriminating understanding). The horses are the *indriyāṇi,* normally rendered "senses" but "life powers" may be more suitable. In present form the indriyani are the senses and instincts. They are of two groups—the five powers of knowing *(jñānendriyāṇi),* namely, the five senses, and the powers of acting, enumerated as the organs of speech, reproduction, evacuation, hands and feet (refering not simply to the organs but to their functions).

As driver, intelligence *(buddhi)* controls the horses (senses and instincts) by means of the mind. *Manas* is the chief organ of the conscious life that shapes into perceptions the impressions of the senses, and also translates these perceptions into conative acts expressed through the organs of action. It is imperative that the mind be controlled by the higher power of reason and intelligence. The person who possesses such a discriminating understanding, controlling the impulses of the mind, which is then said to be yoked *(yukta)*, is called wise *(vijñānavan)*, a person of right understanding; while the individual lacking such such a discriminating controlling judgment, whose mind is therefore unyoked *(ayukta)*, is dubbed without understanding *(avijñānavan)*. A controlling understanding makes a person attentive and steady-minded *(samanaska)*, otherwise the mind is inattentive and shifty *(amanaska)*. It is impossible for a mind in this unstable state to control the senses and instincts, which cut loose like wild horses.

A second important theoretical account of the origin of *āyus* bears the influence of Sāṁkhya philosophy. This is not the place to give an exposition of Sāṁkhya, but only to highlight elements of the system that have bearing on the presuppositions of Āyurveda. First we highlight the Sāṁkhya theory of causation *(satkārya-vāda)*. This theory postulates that an effect originally exists in its material cause prior to its appearance as an effect. Thus, the pot exists implicitly in the clay; the oil in the seed; and the curd in the milk. The logical consequence of the doctrine of *satkārya-vāda* is that *prakṛti* (material ground) is the ultimate cause of all objects of the material world, including the human mind, intellect, body, and senses. Sāṁkhya is a dualistic system in which *prakṛti* is the material principle. As the uncaused cause of all that is, *prakṛti* is eternal, subtle, and universally pervasive. Its existence as the ultimate ground of the world is inferred by various logical reasons.

Prakṛti is composed of three elements: *sattva, rajas, and tamas*, which are inferred as existing in the ultimate cause by an examination of the ordinary objects of the world. They are the elements of pleasure, pain, and indifference, respectively, and are called *guṇas* because they serve the ends of *puruṣa*, the second ultimate principle. *Sattva guṇa* is the inherent power in people and things that makes for happiness, lightness, and illumination. *Rajas guṇa* is the power of mobility, which gives rise to the experiences of pain. It is the driving force of *sattva* and *tamas*, which, by themselves, are motionless. *Tamas guṇa* is the power of indifference; it produces ignorance, resistance, and confusion. The guṇas are inherently opposed to one another, and yet cooperate in the functioning of all objects in the world. The degree to which one *guṇa* prevails over the other two determines the nature of that person or thing. This does not imply a condition of stasis, for all things in the world are continuously in process due to the volatile character of the *guṇas;* however, a distinction is made in the states of cosmic dissolution and evolution. Before creation *(pralaya),* the *guṇas* change internally and homogeneously, and in the absence of combinations, cosmic equilibrium prevails *(saṁyavastha).* The creative process begins once the *guṇas* interact with one another; this heterogeneous transformation is known as *virūpa-parināma.*

The second principle in this dualistic system is *puruṣa* or the Self. *Puruṣa* is the pure, eternal, all-pervading consciousness. In the individual, the self is a conscious spirit and is to be distinguished from the total body-mind complex. At all times it is the subject of knowledge—never the object.

Evolution commences when nonintelligent *prakṛti* comes into contact *(saṁyoga)* with inactive *puruṣa.* The contact serves mutual purposes, analogous to the cooperation of a blind man and lame man, trying to make their way out of a forest. The encounter shatters cosmic equilibrium, and the activated *guṇas* contend with each other for predominance, combining in varied strengths, and thereby producing different objects in the world. The first product of *prakṛti* is *mahat* or *buddhi.* In the macrocosmos, it is cosmic intelligence *(mahat);* in the individual, it is intellect *(buddhi).* Intellect has closest affinity to the transcendent, and in its pure *(sattvika)* state enjoys health and happiness; but vitiated by *tamas*, it becomes the ignorant prey of sorrow and disease. The second product of *prakṛti* is ego *(ahaṅkāra),* the sense of "mineness." From the *sattvik* side of ego evolve the five organs of perception, the five organs of action, and the mind *(manas).* From the *tamasik* side of ego, the five subtle elements are derived, called *tanmātras.* The *rajas* side of ego supplies the energy for the transformation of *sattva* and *tamas* into their evolutes.

This sketch of Sāṁkhya should suffice to bring out important medical implications.

First, there are the two ultimate principles, *puruṣa* and *prakṛti*, which, though opposite, nevertheless cooperate with one another in the act of creation.

This cooperation among opposites is also evident in the functioning of the four components of *Āyus*, which are further divided into the following twelve factors:

- *Śarīra*—(1) *Vāta;* (2) *Pitta;* (3) *Kapha*
- *Indriya*—(1) Auditory; (2) Tactile; (3); (4) Gustatory; (5) Olfactory
- *Sattva*—(1) *Sattva;* (2) *Rajas;* (3) *Tamas*
- *Ātman*—Consciousness[39]

Some scholars define *Āyus* as "Combination of Śarīr and Prāṇa," but we prefer P. V. Sharma's definition of *Āyus* as "Combination of *Prāṇas*." This definition has the merit of bringing out the cooperation between opposite components in the functioning of *Āyus*.

For closer analysis of the harmonizing activity of these twelve components of Āyus, we segregate the third factor (*Sattva*), involving the three modes of nature: sattva ("subtle matter of pure thought"); *rajas* ("kinetic matter of pure energy"); and *tamas* ("reified matter of inertia").[40] Just as in the case of a lamp, the ingredients of fire, oil, and wick, though possessed of mutually inhibiting properties, function together to produce light; so, too, the three diverse dispositions of nature harmonize to enable the human spirit to become enlightened and thereby achieve liberation.

Thus, for Āyurveda, spirit and matter, soul and body, although different, are not alien, insofar as they can be brought together in a healing relationship with consequences that are mutually beneficial. This is a healthy corrective to the prevailing polarity in medical theory or practice that assumes a mind/body duality.

A second medical implication of the philosophic notion of the unity of the person provides a foundation for the theory and practice of holistic medicine. Theoretically, the *prāṇas* can be isolated from one another, but in the operation of *āyus* this is not possible. Similarly, medical specializtion may warrant the physician to disect a single organ, but that organ never stands alone. The part is only a part of the whole, and is never apart.

The call for integrated medicine is also a call for integrated morality. The "good," for Āyurveda, is always the good for the whole person. In a dilemmatic situation, this could mean, among other things, that efforts to keep the *śarīr* (body) and *indriya* (senses) alive, independently of considerations of the *manas*, *buddhi*, and *ātman*, might prove more heroic than helpful.

On the subject of "holistic" medicine, Larson advances the intriguing notion that this type of Āyurvedic medicine possesses the possibility of encompassing more than one life. In his words:

> Āyurveda assumes that we are much more than a genetic heritage of father and mother. We possess in addition psychic components that may reach back over many lives and may be projected many lives hence. Āyurveda, of course, uses the traditional South Asian idiom for talking about a holistic medicine that encompasses more than one life (in terms of karman, rebirth, transmigration, and so forth). One wonders, however, if it might be possible to translate this ancient idiom into a modern format for research and

study. If such could be accomplished, we might be surprised at the new vistas for philosophical anthropology that would be opened, and we might be surprised to discover that in an important sense the ancient wisdom of traditional South Asian culture has been quietly waiting to be "reborn" and to reveal again its mysteries to us.[41]

Lastly, by espousing the Sāṁkhya philosophy of cosmic evolution, Āyurveda conceives of man in the universe as a microcosm. All forms of matter, including human beings, are composed of five elements: earth, water, fire, air, space. The parallelism between human nature and nature at-large suggests that humans are in a systemic relationship with the creative forces of the universe and encompass powers that are mistakenly attributed to the phenomena of "miracles." For Āyurveda, miracle is not the product of *mantra,* but of *manas*, which can yoke itself to currents of energy that pervade space and time.

This carries us from the philosophies of Vaiśeṣika and Sāṁkhya to the philosophy of Yoga. The Yoga system of Patañjali is closely allied with the Sāṁkhya system. Actually, the spiritual, mental, and physical value of Yoga have been tried and tested in India from the time of the Indus Valley civilization, and it is recognized through all of the subsequent literature. Its contribution in the present context of bioethics is that while it agrees with Sāṁkhya that knowledge of the self's transcendence over the physical world (including the world of our own body, senses, mind, intellect, and ego) is what brings about liberation, such saving knowledge presupposes the purification of the mind and body. The way to this purification is through Yoga. Yoga helps one tune out the whole physical world in which one is normally enveloped and with which one is prone to identify; what remains is pure self-consciousness. The transcendent spirit is then totally isolated from physical reality and thereby comes into its own—free from all the pain, misery, and death that characterize physical existence. Before we explain the discipline whereby the self is able to distinguish itself from the psycho-physical organism, we need to understand certain fundamentals of Yoga psychology.

First, there is the self *(jīva),* the free spirit that is beyond all physical and psychical changes. This self is associated with the gross body (and particularly with the subtle body comprising the senses), the mind *(manas),* the ego, and the intellect.

The intellect or *citta* (Sāṁkhya—*buddhi*), assumes the forms of various objects through which knowledge arises. For example, our knowledge of a chair is conveyed to us through a mental image of the chair, and that image is due to *citta's* assumption of the form of the chair. Because of this cognitive process, *citta* is in a state of constant change. These changes of *citta* are reflected upon the self due to their association. So it appears that the self *(puruṣa)* suffers change and is subject to disease, decay, and death. In fact, all pain and joy are happenings within the physical and psychical organism of the individual that *puruṣa* transcends; but as long as the changes of citta occur, *puruṣa* will be identified with them.

The unequivocal way of ending this erroneous identification is first by restraining the activities of the body and *citta*, and, finally, by eliminating them. This involves the transmutation of *citta* from its phenomenal state of activity to its original state of nonactivity. Here, precisely, lies the goal of Yoga, and this is what gives it its definition as the "elimination of mental modifications." To achieve this goal, one must climb five levels of the mental life *(cittabhūmi)*. At the fourth level *(ekāgra)*, the mind is freed from all disturbances and can engage in prolonged concentration. But the mental processes are not yet eliminated, and so one advances to the final level *(niruddha)*. Here the mental processes are altogether arrested. The mind returns to its original tranquil state, and the self *(puruṣa)* abides in its own essence. This is true liberation. It marks the end of all pain and suffering. Thus Yoga is a spiritual path, directed toward the total extinction of all pain and misery by means of realizing the self's distinction from the body, the mind and the individual ego.[42]

Building on this description of Yoga psychology, Yoga ethics provides practical methods of purification whereby the self discovers its distinction. The underlying thought is that unless a person is moraly strong, he or she cannot undertake spiritual discipline. Moral integrity is the oxygen for the upward climb.

The Yogic discipline of purification has eight steps (*aṣṭāṅga* Yoga).[42] The first two, *Yama* and *Niyama*, are sensitive to the quality of life style. Inasmuch as the body and mind are in close union, for better or for worse, they are bound to have mutual impact on one another.

The third step, *Āsana*, deals with postures. These are exercises intended to restore the body to high levels of energy due to Yoga's perceived correlation between one's capacity for concentration and one's state of health. Concentration is not just a matter of the mind, but of the body as well. Disease is not only a physical liability, but also a mental and spiritual burden. Various postures are prescribed for every type of ailment. For example, in the case of the *vāta* type of constipation, the recommended *āsanas* are "Backward Bend," "Yoga Mudra," "Knee to Chest,"

"Shoulder Stand," and "Corpse." The *asanas* for the *pitta* type of migraine headache are "Sheetali," "Shoulder Stand," and "Fish." The *asanas* to be performed for sinus congestion are "Fish," "Boat," "Plough," "Bow," and "Breath of Fire."[44]

The fourth step is *Prāṇayāma* or control of breath. This involves the suspension of breathing either in exhalation or inhalation. When this takes place, the capacity for concentration is enhanced. In *Prāṇayāma*, the final purpose is mental, but this exercise also has therapeutic physical effects because the heart is strengthened through respiratory control. The result is similar to that of aerobic exercise, which strengthened the heart to the point that its beat is markedly reduced.

The next three steps are internal to Yoga, as compared with the five previous ones that were external aids. They are *Dhāraṇā, Dhyāna*, and *Samādhi.* These are techniques of concentration whereby one can control the mind without use of the body. They climax in the state of *Samādhi*, in which the subject is lost in the object of contemplation and is therefore not aware of it. *Samādhi* is a difficult state to achieve, requiring years of effort, but in the meantime the *yogin* develops enormous physical and psychic powers that keep the body vital, the mind tranquil, and ensure longevity.

Our brief discussion brings out a distinct correlation between Āyurveda and the science of Yoga. In its goal to isolate spirit from matter, Yoga relies on its mental and physical discipline. It is at this juncture that it makes alliance with Āyurveda, for it is only a fit body that can reach the spiritual goal. At the same time, the physical science of Āyurveda is given direction by the philosophical and psychological insights of Yoga. This mutuality explains why, traditionally, the student of Yoga is first initiated into the study of Āyurveda. For the rest of the Yogi's life, he or she continues to rely upon Āyurveda to maintain stamina. Vasant Lad aptly refers to Āyurveda and Yoga as "sister sciences," and explains why:

> Yoga is the science of union with the Ultimate Being. Āyurveda is the science of living, of daily life. When yogis perform certain postures and follow certain disciplines, they open up and move energies that have accumulated and stagnated in the energy centers. When stagnant, these energies create various ailments. Yogis may temporarily suffer physical and psychological disorder because in the course of yogic cleansing of the mind, body and consciousness, disease-producing toxins are released. Employing Ayurvedic diagnoses and treatments, the yogis deal effectively with these disorders.[45]

Ethics

The issues of freedom and determinism are problematic for all systems of ethics, sacred or secular. In the Hindu tradition the subject appears in the form of the doctrine of karma. Mitchell G. Weiss observes that the study of karma in Āyurveda "shows how conflict between fatalistic aspects of an indigenous traditional concept must be reconciled with a practical system which necessarily assumes that the course of many human ills is not predetermined."[46] Caraka tackles the problem in the areas of embryology and the etiology of specific diseases.

Caraka states that a long and happy life is dependent on the coordination of two factors: *daiva* and *puruṣakara*. *Daiva* is the deed done by oneself in a prior incarnation; and *puruṣakara* is a person's action done here. In both these deeds there are grades of strength and weakness. Deeds are of three types: inferior, medium, and superior. "Coordination of both *daiva* and *puruṣakara* of the superior type is the cause of long, happy and determined life-span, while that of the inferior type is the cause of the contrary."[47] Weak *daiva* is subdued by stronger *puruṣakara*, and stronger *daiva* subdues weak *puruṣakara*.

This means that if somebody has a congenital infirmity due to bad karma in a previous incarnation *(daiva)*, and if he does something medically good about it *(puruṣakara)*, he can offset the severity of the ailment, and have a happy life. The opposite is also true. The formula, therefore, for happiness is to match noble *karman* performed in a previous life *(daiva)* with noble *karman (puruṣakara)* done here and now. On the other hand, if both actions are base, unhappiness will follow in kind; and if both are moderate, life will be moderate.[48]

Caraka vehemently argues with a wealth of imagery against those who believe that the length of our days are somehow sealed in a book of life. Belief in predeterminism must issue in passive behavior. One need not do anything to escape the violent acts of nature, man, or beasts. Having no fear of untimely death, one would do nothing to avoid it. With a keen eye to observation, Caraka unravels the folly of this line of thought.

> If all life spans were fixed, then in search of good health none would employ efficacious remedies or verses, herbs, stones, amulets, bali offerings, oblations, observances, expiations, fasting, benedictions, and prostrations. There would be no disturbed, ferocious, or ill-mannered cattle, elephants, camels, donkeys, horses, buffalos and the like, and nothing such as polluted winds to be avoided. No anxiety about falling from mountains or rough impassable waters; and none whose minds were negligent, insane, disturbed,

fierce, ill-mannered, foolish, avaricious, and lowborn; no enemies, no raging fires, and none of the various poisonous creepers and snakes; no violent acts, no actions out of place or untimely, no kingly wrath. For the occurrence of these and the like would not cause death if the term of all life were fixed and predetermined. Also, the fear of untimely death would not beset those creatures who did not practice the means for fending off fear of untimely death. Undertaking to employ the stories and thoughts of the great seers regarding the prolongation of life would be senseless. Even Indra could not slay with his thunderbolt an enemy whose lifespan was fixed; even the Aśvins [divine physicians] could not comfort with their medicines one who suffers; the great seers could not attain their desired life span by means of austerities; and the great seers together with the lords of the gods who know all that is to be known could not see, teach, nor perform in full measure.

Furthermore, it is our power of observation that is first and foremost of all that is known, and it is by observing that we perceive the following: over the course of great many battles, the life spans of the thousands of men who fight compared with those who do not is not the same; similarly for those who treat every medical condition that may arise versus those who do not. There is also a discrepancy in the life span of those who imbibe poison and those who do not. Jugs for drinking water and ornamental jugs do not last the same amount of time; consequently, duration of life is based on salutary practices, and from the antithesis there is death. Also, dealing in the appropriate manner with adverse geographic locale, season, and one's own characterisitics; dealing with karma and spoiled foods, avoiding over-indulgence, abstinence, or the wrong use of all things, keeping all over-indulgence in check and doing away with lack of restraint, avoiding vagabonds and haste—we perceive that proper regard for these will bring about freedom from disease. On the one hand we observe it and on the other we teach it.[49]

If indeed the days of our lives are not predetermined, the question arises as to what are we to make of the conventional distinction of timely and untimely death. This was the question of Agniveśa to his teacher, and Ātreya responds by comparing a person's life span with an axle:

An axle fitted in a vehicle which is endowed with all the natural qualities carries on and perishes in time by depreciation of its normal limit; similarly, the life-span in a body of a person having a strong constitution and managed properly gets its end and loss of its normal limit. Such death is (known as) timely. (On the other hand), the same axle gets destroyed in the way due to overload, uneven road, want of a road, breaking of wheels, defects in vehicle or driver, separation of the bolt, non-lubrication. . . . [Similarly] the life span comes to an end in the middle due to overexertion, diet not in accordance with *agni*, irregular meals, complicated body postures, over-indulgence in sexual intercourse, company of ignoble persons, suppression of impelled urges, non-suppression of suppresable urges, infliction with

> organisms, poisonous winds and fire, injury and avoidance of food and medicaments, such death is (known as) untimely. Moreover, the death occurred in cases of fever etc. due to faulty management is also untimely.[50]

Weiss correctly observes that "by shifting the emphais of etiology from previous lives to the present, Caraka effectively redefines aspects of an immutable karma doctrine as mutable."[51] The tradition held that ordinarily a person reaps the fruit of actions performed in a previous lifetime, along with the consequences of deeds that are excessively good or bad, and that the ripened fruit of deeds performed in the present existence sets the pattern of future birth, its duration, and types of experiences. However, in Caraka only the fruit of extreme evil cannot be arrested by good deeds in the present. Dasgupta describes Caraka's position as a "common-sense eclecticism" which is unique in Indian philosophy. He explains:

> The fruits of all ordinary actions can be arrested by normal physical ways of well-balanced conduct, the administration of proper medicines and the like. This implies that our ordinary non-moral actions in the proper care of health, taking proper tonics, medicines and the like, can modify or arrest the ordinary course of the fruition of our karma. Thus, according to the effects of my ordinary karma I may have fallen ill; but, if I take due care I may avoid such effects and may still be in good health. According to other theories the law of karma is immutable. Only the fruits of unripe karma can be destroyed by true knowledge. The fruit of ripe karma have to be experienced in any case, even if true knowledge is attained. The peculiar features of Caraka's theory consist in this that he does not introduce this immutability to ripe karmas. The effects of all karmas, excepting those which are extremely strong, can be modified by an apparently non-moral course of conduct, involving the observance of the ordinary daily duties of life.[52]

The average person in the street does not believe in an absolute fatality. He strives toward his goal in the hope that he will eventually succeed. He capitulates to "fate" or "destiny" only when he has come to the end of his rope and there is nothing more that can humanly be done. This common-sense view seems to correspond with Caraka's theory. However, if this is the case, how can the immutability of the law of karma be preserved? In Dasgupta's analysis, "Caraka thinks that it is only the extremely good or bad deeds that have this immutable character. All other effects of ordinary actions can be modified or combated by our efforts. Virtue and vice are not vague and mysterious principles in Caraka, and the separation that appears elsewhere between the moral and the physical sides of an action is not found in his teachings."[53]

Thus, by making a case for the mutability of the law of karma, Caraka opens a window for ethical action. We can preserve and prolong mental and physical health, and keep our senses in control (*indriya-vijaya*) by making intelligent choices, doing things in moderation, and making wise use of medicine. He sums it all up: "One who follows the code of conduct for the healthy, lives a life of hundred years without any abnormality. Such person, praised by the noble ones, fills up the human world with his fame, acquires virtue and wealth, earns friendship of all living beings and at the end, that with holy acts, gets into the virtuous other world. Hence this code should be followed always by all."[54]

With the window open for voluntaristic activity, Caraka says the prime obligation of freedom is: "to thine own self be true." Each person has three desires: for life; for wealth; and for the other world (liberation).[55]

"Out of all these desires, one should follow the desire to live first."[56] Why? Because when life goes, everything goes. Life can be maintained when the healthy person keeps himself healthy, and the sick person seeks medical aid.[56] We note that these two endeavors constitute the twofold aim of Āyurveda, and thereby define its overarching understanding of the "good." Whatever tends toward health is good, and whatever alleviates illness is also good.

With health in place, one should pursue the desire for wealth. "Next to life, it is wealth which is to be sought. There is nothing more sinful than to have a long life without means (of sustenance). Hence one should make effort to achieve these means."[57] Clearly, for Caraka, money is not the root of all evil, but the root of all good. Wealth is an excellent thing because it means power *(artha)*—power primarily for not having to depend on others for support (vs. 5a). The means to wealth is work—"agriculture, animal husbandry, trade, commerce, etc." Work is well-being. Labor is livelihood and long life (vs. 5b). There is no hint here of hereditary wealth, which is in reality a premium paid to idleness, and, in Caraka's book, a sure prescription for ailments of body and mind.

For all his emphasis on wealth, *āyus* is not reduced to economics: "one should pursue the third desire for the other world."[58] He acknowledges this is not self-evident, and therefore some succumb to skepticism while others find refuge in scriptural authoritarianism. Instead, Caraka attempts to establish belief in rebirth by all four means of correct knowledge: "authoritative statement, perception, inference and rationale."[59]

While rebirth postulates life after death, the ultimate goal is to end it because *saṁsāra* is a source of suffering. Freedom, finally, is freedom from *saṁsāra*. Ignorantly we ascribe immortality to our mortal bodies. The body, with which we falsely identify ourselves, must one day perish, and our true self (the *Puruṣa* within) departs, only to be reborn. The great seers viewed this "coming" and "going" in a neverending sea of change as suffering, because it involved repeated separation of the self from the Self. *Saṁsāra* as a form of ontological suffering expands our conventional notions of suffering, and supplies new dimensions to the discussion on the meaning of life and death.

Physiology

Ayurvedic physiology comprises the notions of (a) the *Pancamahābhūtas* (five basic elements); (b) the *Tridoṣas* (three humors); (c) the *Sapta Dhātus* (seven basic tissues); (d) the Thirteen *Agnis* (fires); and (e) the three *Malas* (excretions).

(a) *Pancamahābhūtas* In the course of evolution, according to Sāṁkhya theory, there emerges from inert matter certain subtle materials *(tanmātras)*, which, although imperceptible, have definite characteristics. They are the "generic essences" of physical energy represented by sound, touch, colour, taste, and smell. When these subtle essences begin to compound, gross matter manifests itself in variegated forms. The production of the five gross physical elements takes place in the following manner. First, the sound energy produces the space element *(ākāśa)*, which has sound quality perceived by the ear. Second, the energy of touch, combined with the movement of space, produces air *(vāyu)*, which has the qualities of sound and touch. Third, the energy of color combining with the energies of sound and touch, produce fire *(agni)*, which has the qualities of sound, touch, and color. Fourth, the energy of taste, in combination with the essences of sound, touch, and color, produce water (*jala*), which has the qualities of sound, touch, color, and taste. Fifth, the energy of smell, combining with all of the above essences, produces Earth *(pṛthivī)*, which incorporates the qualities of sound, touch, color, taste, and smell. The subsequent evolution of the world, including the human constitution, is from these five elementary principles of Space, Air, Fire, Water, and Earth. One should not attribute commonplace meanings to these elemental substances.

The five elements enter the body through food and become reconstituted in the physiology and anatomy of the individual. As with the rest of nature, the body is in a continuous state of transformation. Death is the final act by which the organism is returned to its original state.

The point of significance for ethical considerations is that the universe and the human body form a river of life that has its source in creation. We are not strangers in a universe that is alien, or, at best, neutral to human projects, but the universe is the very womb from whence we have come. This understanding of our place in the universe has important implications for how we relate to our bodies, to "proper" foods and drugs, to animal life, and to sun and soil. The bottom line is: the universe, and all of us in it, is *pancamahabhūtika* (of five basic elements).

(b) *The Tridoṣas* The *pancamahabhūtas* take form in the body as the *tridoṣas*, or humors. These three elements are wind *(vāta)*, bile *(pitta)*, and phlegm *(kapha)*. *Vāta* is a product of Space and Air. *Pitta* is produced from Fire and Water; and *kapha* from Earth and Water. These three body elements, along with blood, sustain the body and regulate the organic and psychic functions. Without them, the body cannot exist. When they are in a state of dynamic equilibrium, the body enjoys health and well-being; but when there is a loss of balance, disease results. Each *doṣa* has three states: aggravation, diminution, and equilibrium. Āyurveda maintains that healing can only proceed upon a sound understanding of the *tridoṣas*.

Wind is the most important of the three humors. It is a combination of the two universal elements of Air and Space. *Vāta* refers to motion. "Bodily air, or *vāta*, may be characterized as the subtle energy that governs biological movements. This biological principle of movement engenders all subtle changes in metabolism."[60] *Vāta* is active in the processes of respiration, circulation, evacuation, and chiefly in the functions of the nervous system. It is principally located in the stomach, small intestines, chest, and in all passages, such as the ears, eyes, nose, throat, rectum, and generative organs. There are five kinds of Air, the most important of which is *Prāṇa vāyu*, or Vital Air. It supports life *(prāṇa)* and is situated in the chest. As long as *vāta* is in a state of equilibrium and is able to flow freely over the body to help it perform its vital functions, there is health; but when it is diminished, weakness sets in and diseases arise in the areas of digestion, respiration, circulation, and voice. Hypertension, paralysis, pain, and stiffness of the limbs, and cardiac dysfunction are common. *Vāta* is usually deranged by excessive physical strain, sleeplessness, and eating the wrong quantity and quality of food.

The second humor is *pitta*, or bile. It literally means heat and is composed of the elements of Fire and Earth. It controls the enzymes and hormones and affects all chemical functions, including digestion and metabolism. Body temperature and the tonality of the skin and eyes come from *pitta*, as do emotional intensity and intellectual acuity. It can be disturbed in some forty ways, causing high temperatures and the incidence of jaundice, urticaria, sleeplessness, sluggishness, and a craving for cooling foods. These derangements are often brought on by the harboring of hostile thoughts and feelings, fatigue, fasting, and eating incorrect foods. *Pitta* is found in organs such as the heart, liver, spleen, and skin, but its center is in the stomach and small intestines.

The third humor is *kapha*, or phlegm. It regulates the two other humors and is a combination of Space and Water. It is chiefly located in the region of the head, chest, stomach and is found in the moist parts of the anatomy. There are five kinds of phlegm that lubricate the moving parts of the body and provide moisture for the brain, eyes, and skin. *Kapha* also aids in digestion by softening the food; it provides sexual energy; it sustains the entire physical organism; and it helps in such mental processes as memory retention. When *kapha* is morbidly diminished, the body loses its liquidity; vessels are hardened; thirst is sharpened; heat is increased; digestion is impaired; the joints are immobilized; and the individual becomes tardy and anorexic. Causes of these derangements include failure to exercise and faulty diet.

Like the mind, the *tridoṣas* permeate the entire organism, but a special division is ascribed to each one. *Kapha* lies above the navel; *pitta* is in the trunk, above the pelvic region; and *vāta* is below the pelvis. The strength of each is regulated by the time of day. In the cool of the morning, phlegm predominates; in the heat of the midday, the effects of bile are strongest; and in the evening, it is the wind that is most felt. The same principle applies to the changing seasons, each having a proness to a particular *doṣa*. The human life cycle is explained in similar terms. In the growing years, *kapha*, which governs the anabolic process of the body, is most active; in maturity, when life takes on a certain stability, *pitta*, which controls the metabolic process of the body, is at the fore; and in the advanced years, when the body begins to decline, *vāta*, governing the catabolic process, is most manifest. For each region of the body there is an elemental angularity that the physician must take into account in making diagnoses or prescribing remedies. The most fundamental particularity of all is the constitution of each individual. Typically, each person has a characteristic constitution—that of *vāta*, *pitta*, and *kapha*. This does not imply the singularity of any one factor, rather its prevalence in consort with the others. For example, a person of *vāta* constitution has a combination of all three *doṣas*, but it is *vāta* that predominates.

The import for ethics in respect to the *tridoṣa* theory mainly lies in viewing the body organismically by not reducing it to any one of its organs; by being sensitive to body-mind connections; and by recognizing the constitutional individuality of each person, both in diagnosis and treatment.

(c) *The Seven Elements* The five proto-elements *(mahābhūtas)* that are responsible for the creation of the entire material world are also present in the seven elements, and, as in the case of the *tridoṣas*, one or two may predominate. These seven constructing elements are known as *dhātus*, meaning: "that which enters into formation of the basic structure of the body as a whole."[61] Therefore, as the basic tissue elements, the *dhātus* constitute the body and support and sustain it. Of special importance is their role in the body's immunological system. They constitute the body's fluids and its hard and soft parts. These seven elements are: plasma *(rasā)*, blood *(rakta)*, flesh *(māṁsa)*, fat *(meda)*, bone *(asthi)*, marrow *(majjā)*, and semen *(śukra)*.

Rasā is the nutritional extract from digested food and provides nourishment for the entire organism. It enters the blood and is transferred successively into the remaining elements. The blood *(rakta)* is responsible for oxygenating the system and conveying nutrients. Flesh *(māṁsa)* and muscle constitute the organs and supply the body with connective strength. Fat *(meda)* proceeds from flesh and is the lubricating element in all bodily parts. Bone *(asthi)* comes from fat and gives the body its skeletal structure. Marrow *(majjā)* fills the bones and, with the nerves, conveys sensory messages. Sperm *(śukra)* originates from marrow and is the reproductive element.

The seven elements are directly influenced by the *tridoṣas*. Therefore, to maintain them in a state of health, it is necessary to follow a good diet, exercise regularly, and thus keep *vāta, pitta*, and *kapha* in proper balance.

The essence of all of these elements is known as *ojas*, meaning power. It gives vitality to all of the tissues and is found throughout the body. In a healthy state, *ojas* gives firmness to the body, a shining color to the skin, and energizes the internal and external organs. In the event it is diminished by hunger, injury, exhaustion, or anxiety, the individual's complexion changes; he or she feels bloated and complains of fatigue and loss of strength. There are three degrees in the diminution of *ojas*; the last terminates in death.

(d) *The Agnis* Health and healing in the Āyurvedic system is intimately connected to food and its proper digestion. This explains the pivotal function of the *agnis*. They act as enzymes in the digestion and absorption of food. There are thirteen *agnis*, the principal one being located in the stomach and the gastrointestinal tract. The literal meaning of *agni* is fire, and *Jatharagni* is "the digestive fire in the stomach." Its task is to break down the intake of food. Next, there are five *bhūtagnis* relative to the five elements. They are the "fire" in the liver. These enzymes "adapt the broken down food into the homologous chyle" and aid in the process whereby "the *mahābhūtic* composition of the broken down food is now made into the same composition as that of the *mahābhūtas* of the body." There are also seven *dhātvagnis*, which are relative to the seven basic tissues *(dhātus)* of the body. These enzymes work on the "cooked" food, synthesizing the various tissue elements.[62]

In the event that the digestive and metabolic functions of biologic fire are impeded, the unprocessed food accumulates in the intestines and proceeds to decompose. This undigested and unassimilated substance is known as *ama*. It is a major factor in the production of endogenous diseases. It blocks the digestive tracts, and when it is chemically transformed into toxins, it enters the bloodstream, causing injury to the internal organs.

(e) *The Three Malas* These secretions *(malas)* that are counted among the constituents of the body include: urine *(mūtra)*, feces *(shakrit)*, and perspiration *(sweda)*. The *malas* are waste products, following the process of digestion; but in the Āyurvedic sysem, these excretions are not exactly waste. For instance, prior to elimination, the solids in the intestinal tract give it support and retain nutrients that are slowly absorbed.

In summary, the human body is the evolutionary product of *prakṛti* (the ultimate ground) through contact with *puruṣa* (the primal self-conscious principle). In this respect it shares a common origin with all material, living, conscious, and unconscious entities. The normal state of the body is one in which all its elements function in balance, including the eleven *indriyas* (five sense organs, five organs of motion, and the mind); the *tridoṣas* (counterparts of the cosmic principles of air, radiant energy, and water); the thirteen *agnis* (digestive "fires"); the three *malas* (excretions); and the seven *dhātus* (elementary materials, e.g., plasma, blood, marrow, etc.). In Āyurveda, balance is synonymous with health. Caraka states that the maintenance of equilibrium is health, and, conversely, that the disturbance of the equilibrium of tissue elements is disease. This brings us to the Āyurvedic practice of medicine.

Medical Practice

The Vaidya

The practice of Indian medicine through professionals is of ancient ancestry, going back to the Vedas where we are introduced to the *bhiṣaj*. In the Āyurvedic literature, the *bhiṣaj* is now known as the *Vaidya*. The term is a development of *vidyā*, or knowledge, which, through its relation with the word Veda, gives it a religious connotation absent in the earlier title. The Arabic word for doctor, *hakim*, is similarly related to *hikmat*, meaning knowledge. By contrast, the English word "doctor" (Latin, *docere*) connotes the physician's communication of knowledge, instead of its acquisition. Thus from the earliest times, the Indian doctor was looked upon as a person of learning, and by the time of Caraka, knowledge took on a specialized connotation, as the *vaidyas* were organized into a recognized profession.[63]

A primary indicator of the professionalization of the *vaidya* is its strict defense of the ethics and practice of the medical profession by shutting out all impostors. There is abundant evidence that there was a large number of itinerant quacks and charlatans who plied their trade like modern "ambulance chasers." It is said, "There are two types of physicians—one, the promoters of vital breath and destroyers of diseases, and the other, promoters of diseases and destroyers of vital breath."[64] The latter wear only "the garb of the physician." Falsely advertising their skills, "they move from place to place in search of preys. They look for patients like bird catchers spreading their nets for the bird in the forest. They malign the skills of the attending physician, posing dexterity in order to hide their ignorance."[65] Unable to alleviate the diseases, they "blame the patient himself for lack of arrangements, nursing and self-control." Should the patient recover (by other means), they take full credit. When the patient is about to die, they flee to some other place in disguise. They avoid the "asssembly of scholars" and parrrot medical formulas they have memorized, "relevantly or irrelevantly." It is preferable "to self-immolate than to be treated by an ignorant (physician)." Hence, "the wise person desiring (long) life and health should not take any medicine administered by an irrational physician (quack)."[66]

If this tirade against "quacks" smacks somewhat of territoriality, it must be admitted that "the medical profession was one which promised rich rewards, both material and spiritual." Ethically the ambitions and aspirations of the system were locked into the established doctrine that there are three values in life, worthy of pursuit: virtue, wealth, and enjoyment.[67]

Admission to the medical studies was open to the three higher stratas of society. Śūdra students could be admitted, provided they had "good character and parentage," but without benefit of the recitation of initiation *mantras*.[68] The motivation for all candidates should be the three values listed earlier, but, in particular, members of the priestly class should study Āyurveda "for welfare of living beings," the warrior class "for their protection," and members of various occupations would study for professional reasons.

> Education was morally structured. According to Caraka, the candidate should be:
>
> Of tender years, born of a good family, possessed of a desire to learn, strength, energy, contentment, character, self-control, a good retentive memory, intellect, courage, purity of mind and body, a simple and clear comprehension, command a clear insight into the things studied. . . . A man of contrary attributes should not be admitted into (the sacred precincts) of medicine.[69]

The rites of formal initiation of a pupil into the science of medicine *(shishyopanayaniya-madhyayam)* were solemn and similar to those for a brahman religious student. After thrice circumambulating the sacred fire, and having invoked the fire god to bear testimony, the preceptor addressed the initiated disciple as follows:

> Thou shalt renounce lust, anger, greed, ignorance, vanity, egotistic feelings, envy, harshness, niggardliness, falsehood, idleness. . . . Thou shalt do what is pleasant and beneficial to me. . . . If I, on the other hand, treat thee unjustly even with thy perfect obedience and in full conformity to the terms agreed upon, may I incur equal sin with thee, and may all my knowledge prove futile.[70]

Equipped with professional skill and knowledge, the disciple was expected to help brāhmins, elders, preceptors, friends, the indigent, the anchorites, the helpless, "without charging for it any remuneration," but he was prohibited from treating "a professional hunter, a fowler, a habitual sinner, or him who has been degraded in life."[71]

The Oath of Initiation

Caraka's "Oath of Initiation" lies at the heart of professional medical ethics in Āyurveda. It has much in common with the ethical bases of the

Hippocratic Oath, such as being totally committed to the good of the patient, but the Indian code has its own unique features. Belief in the doctrine of karma makes for significant difference. Other features include the obligation to celibacy, abstention from eating meat, bearing arms, causing another's death, and witholding medical assistance from those who oppose the social and political order. The translation of the text we present is by A. Menon and H. F. Haberman. The Oath reads:

1. The teacher should then instruct the disciple in the presence of the sacred fire, Brāhṃaṇas [Brahmins] and physicians.
2. [saying] "Thou shalt lead the life of a celibate, grow thy hair and beard, speak only the truth, eat no meat, eat only pure articles of food, be free from envy and carry no arms.
3. There shall be nothing that thou should not do at my behest except hating the king, causing another's death or committing an act of great unrighteousness or acts leading to calamity.
4. Thou shalt dedicate thyself to me and regard me as thy chief. Thou shalt be subject to me and conduct thyself for my welfare and pleasure. Thou shalt serve and dwell with me like a son or a slave or a supplicant. Thou shalt behave and act without arrogance, with care and attention and with undistracted mind, humility, constant reflection, and ungrudging obedience. Acting either at my behest or otherwise, thou shalt conduct thyself for the achievement of thy teacher's purposes alone, to the best of thy abilities.
5. If thou desirest success, wealth, and fame as a physician and heaven after death, thou shalt pray for the welfare of all creatures beginning with the cows and Brāhṃaṇas.
6. Day and night, however thou mayest be engaged, thou shalt endeavor for the relief of patients with all thy heart and soul. Thou shalt not desert or injure thy patient for the sake of thy life or thy living. Thou shalt not commit adultery even in thought. Even so thou shalt not covet others' possessions. Thou shalt be modest in thy attire and appearance. Thou shouldst not be a drunkard or a sinful man nor shouldst thou associate with the abettors of crimes. Thou shouldst speak words that are gentle, pure and righteous, pleasing, worthy, true, wholesome, and moderate. Thy behavior must be in consideration of time and place and heedful of past experience. Thou shalt act always with a view to the acquisition of knowledge and fullness of equipment.

7. No persons, who are hated by the king or who are haters of the king or who are hated by the public or who are haters of the public, shall receive treatment. Similarly, those who are extremely abnormal, wicked, and of miserable character and conduct, those who have not vindicated their honor, those who are on the point of death, and similarly women who are unattended by their husbands or guardians shall not receive treatment.
8. No offerings of presents by a woman without the behest of her husband or guardian shall be accepted by thee. While entering the patient's house, thou shalt be accompanied by a man who has permission to enter; and thou shalt be well-clad, bent of head, self-possessed and conduct thyself only after repeated consideration. Thou shalt thus properly make thy entry. Having entered, thy speech, mind, intellect, and sense shall be entirely devoted to no other thought than that of being helpful to the patient and of things concerning only him. The peculiar customs of the patient's household shall not be made public. Even knowing that the patient's span of life has come to its close, it shall not be mentioned by thee there, where if so done, it would cause shock to the patient or to others.

   Though possessed of knowledge one should not boast very much of one's knowledge. Most people are offended by the boastfulness of even those who are otherwise good and authoritative.
9. There is no limit at all to the Science of Life, Medicine. So thou shouldst apply thyself to it with diligence. This is how thou shouldst act. Also thou shouldst learn the skill of practice from another without carping. The entire world is the teacher to the intelligent and the foe to the unintelligent. Hence, knowing this well, thou shouldst listen and act according to the words of instruction of even an unfriendly person, when his words are worthy and of a kind as to bring to you fame, long life, strength, and prosperity.
10. Thereafter the teacher should say this—"Thou shouldst conduct thyself properly with the gods, sacred fire, Brāhmaṇas, the guru, the aged, the scholars and the preceptors. If thou hast conducted thyself well with them, the precious stones, the grains and the gods become well disposed toward thee. If thou shouldst conduct thyself otherwise, they become unfavourable to thee." To the teacher who has spoken thus, the disciple should say, "Amen."[72]

The formulation and pursuit of these high standards, without resort to force, must be seen as the by-product of the student-mentor relationship, which Murthy describes as "intimate and affectionate, yet rigid and disciplined."[73] Though paternalistic by Western standards, the "moral and noble behavior of the teacher molded the novice into an efficient physician." Zimmer underlines the effectiveness of this model. He says:

> In its use of this method, Hindu medicine shows its kinship to all other crafts. All varieties of accomplishment in India conform to the inspiring model set up by Brahmin priestcraft in antiquity, which has as its aim the transformation of an ordinary boy. . . . In attaining any sort of skill . . . there is left some secret of real mastership and success which is not to be attained through textbooks or class-training, but must be taken in through a kind of magical union through which the master and pupil become one.[74]

The strength of the master-pupil relationship, to be passed on through the generations, is what invests Caraka's Oath with lasting valididity. Murthy's evaluation is well-made: "This oath not only bears valid testimony to the high level of professional ethics in ancient India but stands preeminently suitable for universal adoption by present day medicine."[75]

Four-Legged Therapeutics

The ethics of teamwork is methodically spelled out in the chapter on the "small quadruple."[76] It describes the "Four-legged Therapeutics," and four qualities of each leg. Medical success is seen as a joint effort in which four agents participate. They are: the "physician, drug, attendant and patient."[77] The role of each is defined by its own "excellence," which is necessary to employ.

The excellence of the physician lies in four professional qualities: "theoretical knowledge, extensive practical experience, dexterity and cleanliness."[78] These qualities enable the physician to grasp "the four aspects"—"cause, symptoms, cure and prevention of diseases." The physician's role is therefore indispensable. "As earth, stick, wheel, thread etc. do not serve the purpose (of making a pitcher) without the potter, the other three legs are in the same position without the physician."[79] One who holds "the honorable degree of 'Vaidya'" is assumed to possess exceptional "learning, rationality, specific knowledge, memory, devotion and action," whereby he "showers happiness on the living beings."[80] In addition to possessing the four qualities, and four aspects of knowledge, the physician is known by four philosophical attitudes—"friendliness and compassion towards the diseased, attachment to the remediable and indifference to those who are moving towards the end."[81]

The second leg of the quadruple is the drug. It must have the following four qualities—"abundance, effectivity, various pharmaceutical forms and normal composition."[82]

The third leg is the attendant. Four qualities he must possess are: "knowledge of attendance, dexterity, loyalty and cleanliness."[83]

The patient is the fourth leg. His or her four qualities are: "memory, obedience, fearlessness and providing all information about the disorder."[84]

Thus, therapeutics in Āyurveda is four-legged and has sixteen qualities, which are a blend of noetic and moral values. It is a participatory effort in which professionals and medications constitute three legs, but the stool would topple without the fourth leg—the patient. In Āyurveda, the Western notion of the *patient* as having the sole excellence of *patience* is a veritable misnomer. Participation, not passivity, is the virtue of the Indian patient.

The Vaidya at Work

Having been duly initiated and admitted into the science of medicine, and upon completion of medical training, the young *vaidya* could commence practicing with permission of the king of his country. He must be clean in habits, well-groomed, and manicured. Attired in white garments, wearing shoes, and carrying a stick and umbrella in his hands, he should make his rounds "with a mild and benignant look as a friend of all created beings, ready to help all, and frank and friendly in his talk and demeanour, and never allowing the full control of his reason or intellectual powers to be in any way disturbed or interfered with."[85]

When he enters the sick room, "the physician should view the body of his patient, touch it with his own hands, and enquire (about his complaint)." He should try to ascertain the nature of the disease by means of oral enquiry, plus the employment of all five of his senses.[86]

The high quality of medical care elicited corresponding trust in patients. "The patient, who may mistrust his own parents, sons and relations, should repose an implicit faith in his own physician, and put his own life into his hands, without the least apprehension of danger." For his part, "a physician should protect his patient as his own begotten son." By doing good to humanity with his medical skill, "a physican achieves glory, and acquires the plaudits of the good and wise in this life, and shall live in Paradise in the next."[87]

Of course, the physician could not survive on plaudits and dream of Paradise; he required adequate compensation for his services. On the one hand, he rendered eleemosynary service to the indigent, but on the other hand he charged handsome fees to those who could afford it. It was not considered unethical to advertise; *vaidyas* walked the streets, asking: "Who is ill here? Whom shall I cure?" Often they could not be distinguished from charlatans who enjoyed festive occassions, because people would eat and drink excessively and develop intestinal problems. Quacks also plied their practice to gain access to female quarters, with an eye to full examination.

As a means toward ensuring high standards of professionalism, a system of royal licensure (*rājānujñāta*) became common practice from early times. By Suśruta's account, "A physician having thoroughly studied the Science of medicine, and fully pondered on and verified the truths he has assimilated, both by observation and practice, and having attained to that stage of (lucid) knowledge, which would enable him to make a clear exposition of the science, should open his medical career . . . with the permission of the king of his country."[88] According to Dalhaṇa, a twelfth-century commentator, the chief intent of the system was to keep out ignorant pretenders to skill in medicine.[89]

The government's stake in public health was based on Hinduism's political ethic that mandated that the primary function of the king was the "protection" of his people. Basham notes that "this function was not taken as the mere protection of life and property from internal and external enemies, but was interpreted in a positive sense."[90] Caraka specifes that Āyurveda should be studied and promoted by royalty "for the purpose of protection" (*ārakṣārtham*). Basham cites a comparable passage in the *Kāsyapa Saṃhitā*, a later text that is dependent on Caraka, in which it is clear that the king was expected to *protect his subjects, not himself.* It is abundantly clear that the king and wealthy members of society considered it their obligatory service to provide medical assistance for persons who did not have the means.

Health and Longevity

Āyurveda has an integrated understanding of health that includes the psyche (*manas*), the *soma* (*śārīra*), and the the *ātma* (soul). Together they form a tripod, which functions well to the degree it maintains a functional balance. Suśruta says that a healthy person is one with "a uniformly healthy digestion," and whose bodily humors are in balance, and in whom "the fundamental fluids course in their normal state and quantity," accompanied by the normal processes of secretion, organic function, and intellection. The operative concept in Suśruta's definition of health is *samya*, meaning balance. The notion of balance arises out of an understanding of the human organism as being created out of fundamental components that have evolved out of *prakṛti*, the Ultimate Ground. These *tattvas* are:

- The eleven *indriyas* (mind, the five sense organs, and the five organs of motion and action)
- The three *doṣas* (counterparts of the three cosmic principles of air, radiant energy, and water)
- The *agni* (digestive fire)
- The *malas* (excretions)
- The *kriyas* ("organic functions, such as sleep, flow of body fluid, elimination")
- The seven *dhātus* (root principles)

When these components are in equilibrium, health exists. The purpose of Āyurveda is to maintain this healthy state of harmony and, when *samya* is threatened by *vaishamya* (imbalance), to restore balance.[91]

Of special concern is the balance of the *tridoshas*, but in broader view health is with reference to the whole person, conceived as a composite of body, mind, and soul. A person may be a fine physical specimen, but if he is mentally or spiritually ill, he is not considered a healthy person. Life is not compartmentalized; therefore health must be defined in terms of its totality.

Further, the constitution of each person is unique, by virtue of its *doṣas*; hence the need to view health as individualized. This is apparent in the makeup of the word meaning health—*swastha. Swa* signifies one's own distinctive constitution.

Health is always a precarious state, because it is constantly subject to disturbing factors in the environment. Āyurveda therefore lays great store in the maintenance of health and the prevention of disease. As stated earlier, Āyurveda is more concerned about keeping the body at a peak level of performance, rather than having to resort to curative remedial measures. To fulfill that goal it emphasizes personal hygiene, the impact of external factors, nutrition and diet, rejuvenation, and public sanitation.

Personal Hygiene and Health

Caraka gives the following instructions to be followed on a daily basis, called *dinacharya* and *ratricharya*:

- Awake before sunrise.
- Answer the calls of nature, and clean excretory organs.
- Brush the teeth with astringent, pungent, and bitter twigs, and apply a dentifrice that is compounded of honey, drugs, salt, oil, and fragrance, to cleanse, deodorize, and sweeten the mouth and breath, and to promote cheerfulness of mind. For similar results, scrape the tongue and gargle with medicated oils.
- Wash the face with cold water and deep-cleansing herbs for prevention of skin-blemishes.
- Apply collyrium to the eyes for stimulating secretions.
- Smoke medicated pipe, eight times a day, to clear the head, remove sleepiness, sharpen the intellect, etc. For some, smoking is contraindicated. Excessive smoking is forbidden.
- Use snuff three times a day in early rains, autumn, and spring.
- Moisten head with unctous substance, daily, to avoid headache, alopecia, greying of hair, and to give the face a pleasant glow, along with sound sleep.
- Saturate ears with oil, daily, to offset hearing disorders, stiffness of back, neck and jaws.
- Massage the entire body—"by using oil massage daily, a person is endowed with pleasant touch, trimmed body parts, and becomes strong, charming and least affected by old age."
- Bathe frequently—it is "a purifying aphrodisiac, life-promoting, destroyer of fatigue, sweat and dirt, resuscitative, and a good promoter of *ojas*."
- Wear clean clothes—it "enhances charm, fame, life span; removes inauspiciouness, produces pleasure, auspiciousness and eligibility for a congregation."
- Use fragrance and garlands as aphrodisiacs, to produce good smell, longevity, charm, nourishment and strength, pleasing manners, and to destroy inauspiciousness.
- Wear gems and ornaments to promote wealth, auspiciousness, longevity, prosperity, happiness, charm, and *ojas*.
- Clean feet and excretory organs frequently to promote intelligence, purity, longevity, and auspiciousness.

- Cut hair, beard, moustache, nails, etc.—good grooming is "nutritive, aphrodisiac, life-promoter, and provides cleanliness and beautification."
- Use footwear—"beneficial for eye-sight and tactile sense-organs, is destroyer of calamity to feet and promotes strength, ease in display of energy and libido."
- Use an umbrella—alleviates "natural calamities, provides strength, protection, covering and well being, and guards against the sun, wind, dust and rains."
- Use a stick—supports balance, averts enemies, gives strength and longevity, and destroys fears.
- Take up those professions that are not contradictory to *dharma* (social and religious ethics). Pursue life of peace and study to achieve happiness.
- Exercise to achieve firmness and strength, but in moderation to avoid fatigue, exhaustion, emaciation, thirst, internal hemorrhage, etc.
- Do not suppress natural urges and bodily functions to urinate, defecate, ejaculate, pass wind, vomit, sneeze, belch, yawn, eat, drink, cry, sleep.
- Suppress "the urges of evil ventures relating to thought, speech and action"—mental impulses are equally harmful to body and mind.[92]

In addition to the daily routine of *dinacharya* and *ratricharya*, Caraka gives preventive health tips to be accommodated to seasonal changes. The year is divided into six parts, with each producing peaks and valleys, high points and hazards for a person's given constitution. Actitivities must therefore be planned around the seasons. For instance, in winter one should eat "sour and salted juice of the meat of dominantly fatty aquatic and marshy animals. . . . drink wine, vinegar and honey. . . . use massage . . . heated rooms . . . use carriages, beds, and seats well-covered . . . clothes should be heavy and warm. . . . While on bed, he should sleep, embracing well-developed women having big and prominent breasts . . . and enjoy sexual intercourse up to full satisfaction at the advent of sisira." But signals change when summer comes. "During summer, one should resort to forests, cold water and flowers, avoiding sexual intercourse altogether."[93] To adjust to these seasonal transitions, three times a year, at set seasons, the body should be cleansed of accumulated wastes through sudation, steam-baths, emesis, laxatives, enemas, and douches.

The ethical component of the many rules on personal hygiene is unmistaken: persons must assume responsibility for the maintenance of their health by taking preventive actions that are medically informed, rationally conceived, practically designed, individually measured, holistically applied, and situationally asessed. Caraka uses the simile of a charioteer and his chariot to make his basic point: As a charioteer is aware of the rules of defensive driving, a wise person should be aware of the duties relating to his own body. In modern metaphor, "Don't drive your car into the ground; follow the "Owner's Manual"; service regularly; and it will give you miles of care-free driving!"

Heredity, Environment, Topography, and Health

Health is conditioned by internal factors, as in the case of personal hygiene; it is also dependent on external factors, such as heredity, environment, and topography.

On heredity, Caraka states that the embryo is an aggregate of several factors, including parents. "The embryo is produced by the mother," and he specifies entities that are derived from the mother. Similarly, "The embryo is produced by the father," and he lists entities that are specifically paternal.[94]

The environment also impinges upon health. Astral and planetary changes affect the seasons, and these atmospheric shifts leave their mark on the quality and quantity of plant life, which, in turn, set the conditions for disease. Further environmental deterioration or derangement in respect to the environmental factors of air, water, place, and time produce epidemics that attack the health of total communities.[95]

Food and Health

Food is one of the six building blocks of life. It is cosmic matter in the form of nutrition. It is the most potent source of health. Along with sleep and self-control, food is one of life's three pillars.

According to the medical texts, you are what you eat, and you must eat what you are. That is, the food you eat should be suited to your individual constitution. This requires a knowledge of your own constitution and an understanding of how it relates to the qualities of diverse foods, depending on whether they help or hinder your doshic balance. This is summed up in Caraka's definition of wholesome and unwholesome food: "The food, which maintains the balanced dhātus in normalcy and restores the equilibrium in mal-balanced ones, should be taken as wholesome"; the opposite is unwholesome.[96]

Food is of two types according to its source: "immobile (plant kingdom) and mobile (animal kingdom)."[97]

Food is of four types according to its way of intake: "drinks, eatables, chewables and likeables."[98]

Food is of twenty types according to properties, such as "heavy-light, cold-hot, unctous-rough, dull-sharp, stable-mobile, soft-hard, non-slimy-slimy, smooth-coarse, minute-gross and viscuous-liquid. It has innumerable variations due to abundance of substances, their combination and preparations."[99]

It is emphasized that one's physical and mental constitution *(prakriti)* can change the character of food we eat—light food can become heavy, and vice versa. A long list of items that are wholesome for most people is supplied.[100]

To be on the safe side, one should have a diet that combines all six tastes—sweet, sour, salty, bitter, pungent, and astringent. The point is, each dietary, medicinal, and herbal substance possesses a specific taste, and when the tastes are utilized proportionately, balance ensues. Moreover, the six tastes correspond to six groups of taste buds on our tongues. Ultimately the six tastes are derived from the five *mahābhūtas*:

- Earth + Water = Sweet
- Earth + Fire = Sour
- Water + Fire = Salty
- Fire + Air = Pungent
- Air = Space = Bitter
- Air = Earth =Astringent

When the tongue tastes something salty or sweet, a signal is relayed to the brain, and from there other signals are emitted that affect the *doṣas*, the cells, tissues, organs, and systems of the whole body.

A person who understands the mechanism whereby the *doṣas* are affected by tastes will exercise dietary good sense, so that a person of *vāta* constitution, for instance, will not eat bitter, pungent, and astringent foods in excess, because he knows they tend to produce flatulence. On the other hand, his constitution is well-suited to foods that are sweet, sour, and salty.

All of this dictates the need for cultivating healthy food habits. The Vimānasthānam prescribes the following:

- Eat warm food—it tastes good, stimulates the digestive fire, is easily digested, carminates flatus, and reduces mucus.
- Eat unctous food—it incorporates all of the above effects, plus it develops the body, firms the sense organs, increases strength, and produces clarity of complexion.
- Eat food in proper quantity—it is digested easily, and passes down into the anus comfortably.
- Eat food only after the previous meal has been digested—it prevents the mixing of foods and the vitiation of the *doṣas, agni* is stimulated, appetite is whetted, entrances to the channels are opened, eructation is pure, the heart is normal, flatus passes down, and urges of urination and evacuation are attended to.
- Eat food consisting of items productive of potency—one avoids disorders caused by substances that are antagonistic to bodily and mental powers.
- Eat food chosen according to the seasons *(ritus)*—healthy foods for winter are not good for spring.
- Eat food in a conducive setting, having a pleasant ambience, and in comfortable dress. Help yourself enjoy eating by putting on some music or setting the table. Focus on the food, free of any unpleasant psychic distraction or disturbance. You will probably eat less, too
- Eat food without gulping it down—eating fast, the food may enter a wrong passage and you will not be able to taste its merits or defects. Teach yourself to eat slowly and really savor your food.
- Eat food, but not as the birds do—one grain at a time. A meal that is too slow and of endless duration does not give satisfaction. You will tend to eat too much; the food will become cold; and will be digested irregularly.
- Eat food while not caught up in conversation (or watching TV)—the distracted mind is afflicted with the same hazards as the one that simply stuffs the food down.
- Eat food with due consideration to yourself—check to see whether the food is best suited to yourself in order to derive full benefits.[101]

The role of digestion is central to each of the above prescriptions. In addition to the titillation of the taste buds, the part played by the mind is equally important: "Even wholesome food taken in proper quantity, does not get digested due to anxiety, grief, fear, and anger."[102]

This brings us to the final point: food not only affects the body but the mind. In addition to our physical constitutions *(vāta-pitta-kapha)*, we possess mental constitutions in terms of *guṇas (sattva-rajas-kapha)*. The Sāṁkhya philosophy of creation asserts that the three *guṇas* are universal qualities, necesary for the creation of the universe. In addition they are essential for the maintenance of our psychobiological functions.

Thus in the Āyurvedic tradition, food and health are synonymous terms inasmuch as the proper use of environmental matter in the form of food is the chief cause of health. Hence all of the minute classifications by taste, properties, modes of cooking, time, place, seasons, constitution, and so on. Food is therefore more than a meal—it is morality. We are obligated to eat wisely and well, because food is directly related to the humors and their equilibrium. Food is the best form of medicine. *Hita-ahara* is not simply picking what happens to be on the menu, or being impelled by urges, but being responsible for wholesome food that makes for a healthy, happy life *(sukha)*. The ethics of *Hita-ahara* is taking food that is good for the body; good for the senses, good for the mind, and good for the soul.

Weight and Health

Caraka states that being overweight and underweight are undesirable features of the body that retard health.[103]

A person is called "over-obese" who, " due to excessive increase of fat and muscles, has pendulous buttocks, abdomen and breasts and suffers from deficient metabolism and energy." The over-obese have eight defects:

- Short lifespan
- Hampered movements
- Difficulty in sexual intercourse
- Debility
- Body odor
- Excessive sweat
- Voracious appetite
- Insatiable thirst[104]

Causes of obesity include "over-saturation, intake of heavy, sweet, cold and fatty diet, indulgence in day-sleeping . . . lack of mental work and genetic defect." The lifespan is shortened because of excessive fat, and because only fat is accumulated in the body and not other *dhātus*. Movements are hampered, because of "laxity, softness and heaviness of fat." Sexual intercourse is difficult due to paucity of semen, and fat covering the organ. Debility is the result of the disequilibrium of the *dhātus*. Body odor is related to fat in the body and profuse perspiration. Sweating is due to "association of medas with kapha, its oozing nature, abundance, heaviness and intolerance to physical exercise." Excessive hunger and thirst follow from "intensified agni [digestion] and abundance of vayu in the belly."[105]

Caraka continues. Due to its obstruction in the passage, "fat moves about abundantly in belly and thus stimulates digestion and absorbs food. Hence the person digests food quickly and desires excessively the intake of food."[106] When there is delay in taking food, the person becomes afflicted with severe disorders. *Agni* and *vāyu* are particulary damaging to this person; they "burn the obese like the forest-fire burning the forest." In the event of excessive increase of fat, *vāyu*, etc. *(doṣas)* suddenly give rise to severe disorders and thus shorten the lifespan of the over-obese individual.[107]

At the opposite end of the spectrum from the over-obese person is the over-lean person.[108] The conditions of both are hazardous to health, but the obese are at greater risk when some disease arises.[109]

Features that make a person over-lean are: "indulgence in rough food and drinks, fasting, little diet, excessive subjection to evacuative therapy, grief, suppression of natural urges, including those of sleep, non-unctous anointing in rough persons, indulgence in bath, constitution, old age, continued disorder and anger."[110]

Moreover, the over-lean person is averse to physical exercise, avoids food and drink, cannot tolerate cold or heat, and has no appetite for sexual intercourse. His condition renders him prone to diseases such as spleen enlargement, cough, emaciation, dyspnoea, gaseous tumors, piles, abdominal diseases, and disorders of the *grahani*.[111]

The over-lean is "the person who has dried up buttocks, abdomen and neck; prominent vascular network; only remnant of skin and bone and with thick nodes."[112] The manuals proceed to prescribe health regimens for both conditions.

A healthy person has a balanced proportion of muscles, compactness, firm organs, which make him resistant to disorders. "The person having balanced musculature has got tolerance for hunger, thirst, the sun, cold and exercise; balanced *agni* [digestion] and normal metabolism."[113]

In order to promote the bulk of the obese, heavy and non-saturating therapy is prescribed, while for promoting the bulk of the lean, the therapy is light and saturating.[114]

Specific recommendations for removing over-obesity include food and drink that alleviate *vāta* and reduce *kapha* and fat; rough, hot, and sharp enemas; rough anointing; and the intake of various root-powders mixed with honey. All of this should be accompanied by a gradual increase of vigils, sexual intercourse, physical exercise, and mental work.

Similarly, recommendations for removing over-leanness include sleep, mental relaxation, sexual intercourse, physical exercise, a cheerful attitude, a diet of fresh cereals, new wine, meat-soup, honey etc., unctous enemas, daily oil massage, wearing fine dress and garlands, and uplifting perfumes. Finally, "one becomes corpulent like a boar by not minding about business, saturating diet and indulgence in sleep."[115]

Sleep and Health

In addition to diet, Caraka counts sleep and self-control among the three pillars of health. When these three are observed properly, and thus the body is supported well by these pillars, "it continues well-endowed with strength, complexion and development."

The pillar of sleep supports everything that goes on in life.[116] It gives rest to body and mind, and is essential in the maintenance of health.

Sleep is produced by a variety of causes, such as tiredness of body and mind, trauma to the head, consequence of disease, but the most natural and beneficial cause of sleep is the arrival of nightfall. Sound sleep for six to eight hours relaxes and reinvigorates body and mind and maintains the balance of the *dhātus*. Getting the right amount of sleep depends, once more, on the individual's constitution and the changing seasons. Day-sleep is recommended for those who are emaciated because of lifestyle, overexertion, digestive problems, injuries, suffering from diarrhea, colic, etc., leanness, exhaustion, sleeplessness, and emotional problems.[117]

Inducements to sleep cover a variety of expedients, such as "massage, anointing, bath, meaty-soup . . . rice with curd, milk, fat, wine, mental ease, pleasant smell and sound, gentle rubbing, saturating drops and paste on eyes, head and face, well-covered bed, comfortable room and proper time."[118]

Finally, Caraka gives a list of types of sleep. They are "caused by tamas, caused by kapha, caused by physical exertion, caused by mental exertion, adventious, as sequel to a disease and normally occurring in night."

Normal night-sleep is rated superior by experts, because it best sustains and supports all creatures. Sleep "caused by tamas is known as the root of sin, while the remaining ones are observed in diseases."[119]

Self-Control and Health

The third pillar is *brahmacarya.* It means living a life of self-control and study that leads to a knowledge of Brahmā (God). Spiritually, it is living a life that is dedicated to God; psychologically, it is being non-attached to one's actions, so as to be freed from the stress and strain of ego-possession. Ultimately it is the removal of the ego that makes liberation possible.

For the ascetic, *brahmacarya* means celibacy; for the householder it signifies keeping sexual activity within marriage, refraining from sex during festival days, and during the wife's menstrual periods. Semen *(shukra)* is the distillation of the six *dhātus*, and is the source *(bīja)* of reproduction; hence the need to preserve it for health of body and mind. This brings us to the connection between sexuality and health.

Sexuality and Health

The connection between sexuality and health in the Indian tradition is immensely complex, having ancient beginnings. According to Kakar:

> Sexuality—whether in the erotic flourishes of Indian art and the Dionysian rituals of its popular religion or in the dramatic combat of Yogis with ascetic longings who seek to conquer and transform it into a spiritual power—has been a perennial preoccupation of Hindu culture. In this resides the reason, puzzling to many non-Indians, why in spirit of the surface resemblances between Jungian concepts and Indian thought, it is Freud rather than Jung who fascinates the Indian mind. Many modern Indian mystics feel compelled, in fact, to discuss Freud's assumptions and conclusions about the vagaries and transfigurations of libido, while they pass over Jung's work with benign indifference.[120]

The Indian notion of sexual sublimation stems from *vīrya*—sexual energy in the form of semen. Physical prowess and mental acuity come from *vīrya*. Sexual energy can move downward in the act of intercourse where it is ejaculated in the physical form of semen, or it can spiral upward to the brain in the subtle form of *ojas*. Kakar explains, "Hindus regard the downward movement of sexual energy and its emission as semen as enervating, a debilitating waste of vitality and essential energy . . . on the other hand, [if] semen is retained, converted into *ojas*, and moved upward by the observance of celibacy, it becomes a source of spiritual life rather than a cause of physical decay. Longevity, creativity, and physical and mental vitality are enhanced by the conservation of semen; memory, will power, inspiration—scientific and artistic—all derive from the observation of celibacy. In fact, if unbroken celibacy in thought, word, and deed can be observed for twelve years, the aspirant will obtain *mokṣa* or 'salvation' spontaneously."[121]

The ethical input of these views of sexuality, inspired by the ascetical ideal, is derived from the equation of sexual passions with creative fires—fires that not only have the capacity to procreate, but to self-create. Health is at its highest when the physical can give birth to the spiritual. For his part, Caraka stays within his role as physician, and dispenses "semen of crocodile" as the best aphrodisiac for the patient in search of an out-of-body experience.[122]

The Mind and Health

Mental health is within the domain of *manas*. The role of the mind is to activate, direct, and coordinate the sensory and motor organs; to reason; to deliberate and to discriminate. Counterparts to the physical *doṣas* of *vāta, pitta,* and *kapha* are the two mental *doṣas*—*rajas* and *tamas*. The *doṣas* are in a perpetual state of competition, each seeking supremacy, and thus giving rise to mental and physical disorders. Granted this interaction, it is imprecise to dub a disease as solely physical or mental. The emotional states of anxiety, fear, anger destabilize the physical *doṣas*, while *vāta, pitta, and kapha* produce mental disorders, such as insanity and epilepsy. A healthy mind therefore depends much on the balance of all *doṣas*, physical and mental. Kakar underscores the fact that "Āyurveda . . . is truly dialogical: body and mind make up a whole simultaneously, not sequentially, each being of equal value (with no claim to superiority). In the ultimate analysis, there is no such thing as "physical" illness; there is only illness."[123]

In order to keep the mental humors in a healthy state, a person must not become the slave of his desires, on the one hand, and should be free from the destructive emotions of anger, fear, and envy, on the other. Neither of these tasks is easy, because desire and repulsion have hidden beginnings. "One root extends down to the prenatal stage, around the third and fourth months of pregnancy. In this period the unfulfilled longings of the mother and her unrelieved fears are said to be transmitted to the newly activated psyche of the fetus, where they are stored and thus create the source of eventual suffering."[124] The second root of desire and repulsion steps back in time to a previous birth, when "unfilled longings and unresolved traumas" enter the fetus as "memory-traces," ultimately to surface, "demanding completion and closure, and thus increase both the mental humors."[125]

Folklores in many cultures have some version of the intriguing theory of Āyurveda, that the mother carries a heavy responsibility during the period of gestation. Modern Western medicine limits this responsibility to the physical level by emphasizing good nutrition, exercise, and so on, but it stops short of the conditioning that takes place between mother and fetus on the psychic level. Given the reality of psychosomatic influence, it appears arbitrary to isolate the emotions of the mother in such a sensitive area of human development. Āyurveda's ethic of fetal care thus extends the adage of "do no harm" beyond the toxification of smoking and doing drugs, to toxic thoughts and toxic feelings on the part of the mother.

Further, if Caraka is correct that the physical and mental *doṣas* are like overlapping plates, which keep shifting with the currents, it is a misnomer to use the exclusive labels of "physical" or "mental" to designate health or disease. It is therefore bad medicine and unethical practice for a doctor knowingly to dismiss the psychic component, just because it is elusive and time-consuming.

Social Conduct and Health

Āyurveda's comprehensive understanding of health includes the social dimension. With Aristotle, Caraka sees humans as social animals. Life in the womb is a microcosm of the larger social world. Positive social relationships make for health and the control of sense organs, therefore Caraka admonishes that "one who desires to promote his own well-being should follow . . . the code of good conduct."[126]

Reverence for the divine is the beginning of good conduct. Next to godliness is cleanliness. One should wash twice a day, clean excretory organs and feet frequently. It is a mark of respect how we present ourselves to others through dress, good grooming, adornment with flowers and fragrance, cheerful countenance, stimulating conversation, and hospitality. Society includes the invisible company of departed forefathers, who must be honored with religious offerings.[127]

Outward behavior must be backed by character. In terms of personal qualities, one should be self-controlled, even-keeled, discriminating, free from anxiety, fearless, modest, courageous. One should not yield to enmity, nor should one be vicious, even to sinners. Respecting privacy and confidentiality, one should not disclose the defects of others, neither should one probe into their private lives. In terms of social qualities, one should be truthful, charitable, hospitable, friendly, compassionate, detached, and dedicated to teachers, scholars, and elders.[128]

Conduct should be guided by good manners and etiquette. It is impolite to laugh loudly in public, to yawn or sneeze with uncovered mouth, and to grind one's teeth. It is improper to release body fluids in front of wind, fire, water, the moon, before brahmanas and preceptors, and to urinate on the road and in crowded places, while eating. It is gauche to break wind in the company of others.[129]

Sexual conduct should honor marriage bonds; husbands should not seek the favors of other women.[130] A woman should not be insulted.[131] A man must not have too much faith in the opposite sex; must not disclose secrets to them; nor endow them with authority.[132] Sexual intercourse should not be engaged in at dusk or dawn, in sacred places, in gardens, on raised platforms, at crossroads, on cremations grounds, at execution sites, near water reservoirs, in temples, and in the house of brahmins. Sexual intercourse is forbidden with a menstruating woman, without the stimulus of aphrodisiacs, without intense erection of the penis, on an empty or full stomach, under the pressure of natural urges, in a state of fatigue or fasting, and without full privacy.[133] Bestiality and masturbation are prohibited; also dalliance with eunuchs and prostitutes, and bouts of drinking and gambling.[134]

The moral note that is struck with these numerous rules of good conduct is that humans are social animals who crave positive social relationships for the sake of physical and mental well-being. When relationships become estranged or abnormal, psychosocial pressures come about, which produce psyschosomatic disorders. As G. P. Dubey observes, "Transgressions and sinful acts are the cause of worries and anxiety, and the cessation of all miseries is the ultimate aim of life. To achieve this end an improved mode of living has been described, so that individuals can prevent themselves from psychosocial stress by wrong actions. The basic idea of a good life is that a life should be so regulated that the body and mind may be free from physical and mental disorders."[135]

"The improved mode of living" Dubey refers to includes socioethical considerations that are present within the definition of Āyurveda itself. *Āyus* is of four types: *hita* (useful) and *ahita* (harmful); *sukha* (happy) and *dukkha* (miserable). The first two types have social meanings, whereas the second types have personal meaning. This suggests that within Āyurveda's core understanding of life, a person is expected to be healthy and happy on a personal level, but since that individual is also, organismically, a social entity, he must become a useful *(hita)* member of society. Thus the emphasis of Āyurveda is not only on the personal health of the individual but also on social medicine, which is concerned with the well-being of all other persons in the community. Such concern is supported by empirical studies that validate the physiology of altruism. A person who thinks more of others than himself and is engaged in good works occupies a state of mind and body that is conducive to high levels of enjoyment and energy. The complete opposite is the case of the hypochondriac, who can think only of his own woes.

Finally, the psychosomatic orientation of Āyurveda comes through in the clever combination of the twofold regimens for the maintenance of good health: *Sadvṛtta* (Rules and Good Conduct) and *Svasthavṛtta* (Personal Hygiene). The first engages the psyche, and the second engages the body. The point for bioethics is that both regimens carry equal weight, and therefore considerations of social morality are as important for the total health of the person as considerations of bacteriological infection.

Revitalization and Health

Caraka divides treatment along two lines: (1) *Promotive*—for the healthy; and (2) *Curative*—for those with disorders.

In the first category are (a) *Rasāyana* (promotive treatment) and (b) *Vājīkaraṇ*a (aphrodisiac treatment)

(a) *Rasāyana Rasāyana* is the seventh clinical discipline of *Aṣṭānga* (eightfold) Āyurveda. It is variously defined in the different manuals, but the core meaning is the same. It is made up of two words—*Rasā* + *Āyana*—which refer to nutrition and its circulation in the body. Rasā is the primary *dhātu* produced after the consumption of food. *Dhātus* are the "constructing elements" responsible for the total somatic structure. Their function is to develop and nourish the body and to maintain the different organs, systems, and vital parts in health. The purport of *Rasāyana* is to improve the quality and quantity of *Rasā*, and, through it, the successive *dhātus*—blood, muscle, fat, bone, marrow and nerves, and reproductive tissue. In addition, *Rasāyana* builds up the body's immunity, sharpens mental agility, and produces vitality.

Given the physiological concepts of Āyurveda, R. H. Singh presumes that a *Rasāyana* agent promotes nutrition through one of three modes and calls this "the *Rasāyana* effect." In his insightful theory, the following takes place:

1. By direct enrichment of the nutritional quality of *Rasā* (Posaka Rasā), that is, the nutrient plasma: A large number of *Rasāyana* agents both drugs and foods physically contain in their bulk high quality of nutrients and as such when administered they are directly added to the pool of nutrition and in turn help in improved tissue nourishment leading to subsequent *Rasāyana* effects. Satavari, dugdha, ghṛta, and so on are few of the examples of *Rasāyanas* acting at the level of *Rasā*.
2. By promoting nutrition through improving the *Agnivyapara*—that is, digestion and metabolism. Several *Rasāyana* drugs are known to promote digestion of food and vitalize the metabolic activity resulting in turn in improved nutritional status at the level of the *dhātus*. *Bhallataka* is an example of *Rasāyanas* acting at the level of *Agni*. Many such *Rasāyanas* act indirectly as anabolizers.
3. By promoting the competence of *Srotas*—that is, the microcirculatory channels in the body leading to better bioavailability of nutrients to the tissues and improved tissue perfusion. This is another mode through which a *Rasāyana* remedy may help in promotion of nutritional status. Guggulu, a *Rasāyana* mentioned with priority by Sarngadhara, is an example of *Rasāyanas* effective at the level of *Srotas*. The recently reported hypolipidemic and antiatherosclerotic activity of Guggulu is in conformity with the *Rasāyana* effect of this drug as per the mode previously described.[136]

Caraka describes the "*Rasāyana* effect" in the following manner:

> From promotive treatment, one attains longevity, memory, intelligence, freedom from disorders, youthful age, excellence of lustre, complexion and voice, optimum strength of physique and sense organs, successful words, respectability and brilliance. *Rasāyana* means the way for attaining excellent *rasā*, etc. *(dhātus)* [137]

Like Caraka, Suśruta devotes four chapters to details of *Rasāyana*. He says:

> A wise physician should (invariably) prescribe some sort of tonic (*Rasāyana*) for his patients in their youth and middle age after having their systems (properly) cleansed by the applications of a *Sneha* and purifying

> remedies (emetics and purgatives). A person whose system has not been (previously) cleansed (*sodhana*) with the proper purifying remedies (emetics and purgatives) should not, in any case, have recourse to such tonics inasmuch as they would fail to produce the wished-for result, just as the application of a dye to a piece of dirty cloth will prove non-effective.[138]

Both Caraka and Suśruta agree on the following actions of *Rasāyana*, as listed by Vaidya H. S. Kasture: *Rasyan* produces longevity.

- It improves memory.
- It cures many chronic diseases.
- Maintains youth.
- Creates excellent luster of skin.
- Produces good voice and complexion *(prabhā)*.
- Increases the strength of body and power of sense organs.
- Increases power of psyche and maintains healthy psychic condition by producing *satva guṇa*.
- Gives social respectability (due to health, wealthy life, and *satva prakriti*). [139]

Caraka asserts that even into their sixties, people can regain their youth and hold on to it for a very long time.

Three requisites must be fulfilled prior to treatment: that the patient be fully focused, and of firm faith; that the treatment be undertaken in medical facilities, which are precisely laid out; and that the patient should remain at all times under the physician's supervision. By the opposite token, persons who lack self-control, are addicted to drugs, and are not motivated, cannot qualify for treatment.[140] Thus ethics and virtuous living are equally important for the development of long life.

There are two types of *Rasāyana*—(1) *Kutipraveshika* and (2) *Vatatapika*.[141]

In the case of *Kutipraveshika*, a special *kuti* or room is built for the patient in some isolated locale, having pleasant environs, free of hazards, and with access to all things necessary. The patient is admitted at an auspicious time. His body is rid of all impurities and toxins through oil massage and sudation, and his mind is also emptied of psychological impurities. Cleansed in body and mind, a rigorous regimen follows, with due consideration to the patient's age, constitution, and suitability.[142] He is kept on a strict diet of light gruel and warm water. He must occupy these quarters for a full ninety days, without any distractions, particularly of the opposite sex. The following *Rasāyana* produce optimum effects:

1. *Brahmā Rasāyana*
2. *Chavan Prasha*
3. *Amalak Rasāyana*
4. *Haritakiyoga*[143]

In the case of *Vatatapika Rasāyana*, similar medicinal specifications are followed, though the individual is permitted to engage in outside activities, without any segregation. It is cheap, convenient, but less effective than *Kutipravesika.*

From the viewpoint of ethics it is worthy of note that *Rasāyana* is not only a mode of drugs and diet, but also moral behavior, which impacts both body and mind. It advocates a code of conduct *(acara)* that includes respect for elders, holding to the truth, "nonviolence, avoiding anger, avoiding indulgence in alchohol, sex, excessive labour, keeping peaceful," humble, kind, studious, self-restrained, sensitive to weather and balanced sleep. Singh comments that an aspirant who lives such a life and practices *Sadacara* achieves the "*Rasāyana* effect," namely, enhanced longevity, immunity, and intellect, without benefit of any drugs toward that end. His assumption is correct that the code of *acara* Rasāyana succeeds in releasing the aspirant of stress while promoting emotional balance "with a pronounced anabolic state" that is productive of health and happiness. [144]

Thus *Rasāyana* therapy replenishes and renews body fluids, recaptures vitality and vigor, sharpens mental faculties, enhances memory, strengthens immunity, destroys existing diseases, and unlocks charm and beauty. Such high levels of spiritual, mental, and physical vitality envisaged in *Rasāyana* therapy make popular notions of health as "the absence of disease" mere caricatures of human potential, even in old age.

(b) *Vājīkaraṇa* In addition to *Rasāyana,* Āyurveda has a second promotive therapy for the revitalization of health among men—*Vājīkaraṇa.* The difference between the two is that whereas *Rasāyana* promotes all the *dhātus*, Vājīkaraṇa specializes in the quality and quantity of semen and sexualy potency.

Vājīkaraṇa is "that which produces lineage of progeny, quick sexual stimulation, enables one to perform sexual acts with women uninterruptedly and vigorously like a horse, makes one charming for the women, promotes corpulence, and infallible and indestructible semen, even in old persons, renders one great, having a number of offsprings, like a sacred tree branched profusely and commanding respect and popularity in society."[145]

'*Vaja*' has the dual meaning of speed and semen. *Vājīraṇa* is therefore that branch of Āyurveda that promotes virility. Of course, the quest for virility was there from earliest times. The Atharva Veda (IV,4) contains charms invoking Indra, controller of bodies, to endow a man with the virility of a horse, mule, ram, and bull to enable him to enjoy the embrace of women. The accompanying ritual practice has a characteristic mixture of pharmaceutical applications along with potent symbolisms. A *mantra* is recited: "Bulls have dug thee up, thou art a bull, O herb! Thou art a bull, full of lusty force; in behalf of a bull we dig thee up, full of lusty force." Decoctions are then made from these plants, mixed with milk; a drawn bow is set on his lap; and the man drinks the herbal potion. Similar rituals are performed while the man sits (suggestively) upon a stake or a pestle!

In Āyurveda, Vedic quest for virility turns from charms to aphrodisiacs or vitalizers. As propounded by Lord Ātreya:

> A conscious person should use aphrodisiacs regularly because virtue, wealth, pleasure and fame depend on it. It also gives rise to male offspring.[146]

Thus *progeny* with *pleasure* are the two products of *Vājīkaraṇa*. It is recommended for men above the age of sixteen and below seventy.

The "foremost aphrodisiac" is an "exhilarating woman." Women are the most pleasure-giving, because the female form is the source of highest human sensations; and "progeny too is dependent on woman." "The woman who is beautiful, youthful, endowed with auspicious features, submissive and trained is regarded as the best aphrodisiac."[147]

Several formulations of aphrodisiacs are mentioned, depending on their ingredients. For example: "This *piṇḍarasā* (solidified meat-soup) is aphrodisiac, nourishing and strength-promoting, and by the use of this, one strengthened and sexually excited like a horse, penetrates the penis fully (into the female organ). In the same way, *piṇḍarasā* may be prepared from peacock, partridge and swan which promotes strength, complexion and voice and by the use of which the man behaves like a bull."[148]

However, "semen gets diminished by old age, anxiety, diseases; reduced by evacuative measures, fasting and sexual indulgence. Even a saturated man does not get potency for sexual acts due to wasting, fear, want of confidence, grief, finding fault with the woman, ignorant of the enjoyment with them, lack of determination and interest, because potency is based on (sexual) exhilaration, which again depends on the strength of body and mind."[149]

We concur with Singh's observation that whereas the Law-Books, such as Manu, have emphasized the procreative aspect of sex, Vātsyāyana and company have celebrated sex as enjoyment. For their part, the medical manuals combine procreation and pleasure, and find intrinsic connections between the two. Sex for *procreation* and sex for *recreation* are not opposites, but Mother Nature's trick of spicing the need for perpetuity with pleasure.

The significance of *Vājīkaraṇa* for healthy sex in our day is that the aphrodisiacs are designed to activate the production of the body's own energies (sex hormones). In addition to strengthening physique, so as to facilitate the body's natural blood flow, and to activate the production of essential components that help to facilitate blood flow to the penis for a strong erection, *Vājīkaraṇa* also draws on the power of the mind and passion that flows from an aroused imagination. When body and mind are thus united, and energy (hormonal) levels are elevated, physiologically, we *now* know that the following occur:

- Gains in both strength and frequency of erections.
- Intensified increase in sex drive
- Greater increases in sperm production
- Less refractory time (the amount of time needed to recover after ejaculation for repeated encounters)
- Erection is sustained for longer periods of performance

Caraka concludes: "By proper use of these formulations one becomes endowed with good physique, potency, strength and complexion, exhilarated and potent for women like an eight year old horse.

Whatever is pleasing to the mind, beautiful landscape, sandy places, hills, favourite women, ornaments, perfumes, garlands and dear friends—all these help in this process."[150]

Public Health

In addition to the ethics of personal hygiene, Āyurveda has a collective ethic of public health. It is aware of public sources of infection, and cautions against contact with places such as garbage dumps, cremation grounds, public baths, and sacrificial sites. People are held responsible for unhygienic public behavior in the form of sneezing without covering the mouth, spitting in walkways, defecating and urinating indiscriminately, having offensive body odor, wearing dirty garments, failing to perform ablutions, eating out of broken dishes, and spreading sexually transmitted diseases. Epidemics strike whole communities.[151] They are caused by defects and derangements in air, water, soil, and season. These may be called "acts of God," but humans are implicated when they fail to clean water that is obviously polluted, because of its odor, color, taste, touch, and is abandoned by aquatic birds and animals which are smart enough to know it is unfit for habitatation. Similarly, when the life of the land is sick, people are responsible for such things as mosquito and fly control, rodent eradication, clearing vegetation that chokes crops, and so on.[152]

The overall strategy against epidemics which affect large communities is public health armed with preventive measures. Caraka says, "Inspite of these epidemic-producing factors being deranged, the persons managed with (preventive) therapy remain immune against the diseases."[153] Thus public health and preventive medicine are synonymous terms in Āyurveda. They represent the best health insurance for a community and are more important than the need for medicine.

Lifestyle and Health

Lifestyle is the living link between all the diverse approaches to health discussed in this section—from food, sleep, sexuality, and self-contol, to social conduct, revitalization, and public health. The evidence is clear: Āyurveda claims there is a *cause/effect relationship between health habits and longevity*. Additionally, because Āyurveda finds a close link between states of mind and body, it nurtures *stress-free mental conditions* in the pursuit of a happy and useful life. Pregnant women are to be especially careful, both for their sakes and for the health of their babies, with respect to their habits of eating and drinking, their modes of conduct, and their emotional life.

Today the preeminence given by Āyurveda to lifestyle as the hallmark of its system of preventive medicine is being validated by scientific data.

Research published in the *Journal of the American Medical Association*[154] states that people who do not smoke and who maintain low cholesterol and blood pressure levels can live about six to nine and a half years longer than those less careful about their health, according to studies of more than 360,000 patients. The research found dramatic, life-extending benefits for adults of all ages who have low heart disease risk factors.

"These findings are relevant for the national effort to end the coronary heart disease—cardio-vascular epidemic," the study says. "For upcoming generations this means encouraging favorable behaviors beginning in early childhood in regard to eating, drinking, exercising and smoking."[155]

It is additionally noteworthy that from among the hundreds of Christian denominations in the United States, national statistics consistently place members of the Mormon Church and the Seventh Day Adventist Church highest in terms of longevity. Upon investigation it soon becomes apparent that this achievement has less to do with theology and more to do with lifestyle. Proof of this is that members of these communities only raised their life expectancy rates when they began emphasizing lifestyle changes in their followers, not before. Today both denominations are respected for their adherence to strict moral lifestyles that forbid sexual promiscuity, the use of drugs, the intake of unwholesome foods and drinks, and risky behaviors.

Disease

Āyurveda generally views disease in obverse terms to health. Having covered the issues of health at some length, we shall be briefer in our remarks on disease.

Āyurveda's integrative understanding of the person is expressed through the metaphor of the tripod, signifying the balance of the body *(śarīra)*, the mind *(manas)*, and soul *(ātma)*. When a person's *doṣas*, *agnis*, *dhātus*, and *malas* are normal in makeup and function, along with the well-being of *ātma* and *manas*, the individual enjoys health. In the moment this balance is upset, pathological deviations produce pain, which may be felt in the body, or mind, or in both. In the description of Aṣṭānga Hṛdyam:

> *Hina* [inadequate], *mithyā* [perverse] and *ati* [excess], *yoga* [association] of *kāla* [season], *artha* [objects of senses] and karma [activities] are the chief causes of disease; whereas their *samyak yoga* [proper association] is the chief cause of health.
>
> *Roga* [disease] is [the effect of] disequilibrium of the *doṣas* while health is [the result of] the equilibrium of the *doṣas*.
>
> *Roga* is said to be of two kinds, *nija* [organic, arising from the body] and *āgañtu* [traumatic, arising from external causes].
>
> Their [of diseases] *adhiṣṭhāna* [seat] is also of two: *kāya* [the body] and *manas* [the mind].[156]

Murthy comments: "Each *doṣa* is endowed with distinguishing quantities, qualities and functions, and their mutual collaboration is known as *sāmya* (equilibrium). When there is any increase *(vṛddhi)* or decrease *(kṣaya)* in terms of quantity, quality or function, a state of *vaiṣamya* (disequilibrium) ensues."[157]

Rajas and *tamas* are *doṣas* of the mind. We note here that *satva, rajas,* and *tamas* are the three *mahāguṇas* or primary qualities responsible for the whole creative process. *Satva* does not feature in disease, because it is pure, but *rajas* and *tamas* do, when they increase beyond specific limits.

The texts classify disease according to (1) therapy, (2) prognosis, (3) locus, and (4) etiology.

(1) Suśruta states: "Diseases may be grouped under two broad subdivisions, such as Surgical, and Medical, that is those that yield to the administration of purgatives, emetics, oils, diaphoretics, and unguents."[158]

(2) In terms of prognosis, diseases are classified as curable by treatment *(sādhya),* incurable by treatment *(asādhya),* and relievable by treatment *(yāpya).*[159]

(3) The locus of the disease may be on the level of the mind *(manas)* or of the body *(śārīra).*

(4) The etiological classification of disease has many forms: (i) *ādhyātmika*—arising from internal physical or psychic causes; (ii) *ādhibhautika*—produced by causes in the "physical and material environment of the body"; (iii) *ādhidaivika*—the result of providential or demonic causes, or of fate.[160]

Ādhyātmika diseases are threefold: those caused by genetic factors, traced to defects in the father's sperm or the mother's ovum *(ādibalapravṛtta);* caused by congenital factors, due to deranged metabolism *(rasakṛta),* or by psychological disturbances, such as "ungratified hankerings, gratification of improper longings or sinful conduct" on the part of the pregnant mother *(janmabalapravṛtta);* caused by humoral disturbance, due to bad conduct or diet, which upset the metabolic processes; and also psychic disorders caused by deranged humours that have been vitiated by imbalances of the *guṇas (doṣabalapravṛtta).*

Ādhibhautika diseases are of two types: traumatic diseases brought about by hard blows, falls, and bites of animals or snakes *(saṃghātabalapravṛtta);* and seasonal diseases, sparked by heat, humidity, etc. *(kālabalapravṛtta).*

Adhidaivika diseases are also of two types: "providential" *(daivabalapravṛtta)* acts that strike individuals, and epidemics that blanket whole communities; and also natural diseases, such as senility, hunger, thirst, sleep, death and so on that take their toll, regardless of one's good or bad behavior *(svabhāvabalapravṛtta).*[161]

Suśruta delineates three stages in the progress of a disease: a preliminary stage, indicating the advent of the primary disease *(anyalakṣaṇa)*; the arrival of the primary disease *(prāk-kevala)*; symptoms proceeding from the primary disease *(aupasargika)*.[162]

The bioethical significance of Āyurveda's understanding of disease lies in its acceptance of the ambiguity of disease as both "given" and "chosen." On the "fate" side of the ledger are the *ādhibhautika* genre of diseases due to the "acts of God," accidents, and changes in the seasons. Such diseases are out of one's control, at least in terms of their origin. Also, for the person affected, there are hereditary factors, as in the cases of diseases classified as *ādibalapravṛtta* and *janmabalapravṛtta*. These are cases in which parents have eaten sour grapes, and now the children's teeth are set on edge.

At the same time, the ethical dimension of disease is not overlooked. True, epidemics come, but the populace can brace itself from maximum destruction by observing the preventive rules of public health. Likewise the father and mother are not faulted for having defective sperm and ovum, but they are responsible for bringing children into the world when they knowingly engage in acts that are harmful to fetal life. This is not eugenics, but the ethics of sensible parenting.

The mother carries the added onus for her role in the period of gestation. Child-bearing is not only bearing a child, but *bearing responsibility* for its quality of life. "Congenital blindness, deafness, dumbness, nasal voice, cretinism, gigantic structure and similar malformations are caused either by deranged metabolism *(rasakṛta)* or by psychological disturbances (ungratified hankerings, gratification of improper longings or sinful conduct) of the pregnant mother."[163]

The concept of *svabhāvabalapravṛtta* or natural diseases recognizes, on the one hand, that life marches toward death; on the other hand, it believes that the downward trend can be reversed to an appreciable extent. On the downside, these natural processes can be precipitated through unhealthy lifestyles, even making young people old before their time. Physiology counts for more than chronology.

The note of preventive medicine is struck again in tracing the three stages of disease. Wisdom lies in nipping things in the bud, and not allowing them to achieve fatalistic proportions. A fire is most easily extinguished when it is but a spark.

The psyche-soma connection allows for a mix of morals and medicine. Emotions such as anger, fear, and envy are not simply morally bad, affecting character, but are physiologically bad, affecting the body.

The most unequivocal note is struck through the notion of *prajñāparādha*, pinpointing volitional transgression as a factor responsible for exciting the *doṣas* that produce pathogenesis. Transgressions are of three types: speech, mind, and body. The excessive use, disuse, and misuse of these actions result directly in ill health.

In the end, disease is the victor. Its price is death, and all must pay that price, but in the ethics of Āyurveda, it is better to pay later than sooner—not death, but premature death is evil.

Clinical Diagnosis and Treatment

Caraka emphasizes the importance of correct diagnosis of a disease. A physician who is adept in diagnosis, who is proficient in the administration of medicines, and who is fully conversant with the dosage of the therapy that differs from locale to locale and from season to season is bound to succeed.

Āyurveda lays down intricate guidelines for the diagnosis of a vast roster of diseases with reference to their etiology, symptoms, and prognosis.

The diagnostic methodology of Caraka is threefold, based on the *pramāṇas* (sources of knowledge). These are *śabda* (authoritative statements), *pratyakṣa* (direct observation), and *anumāna* (inference).

Authoritative instructions are the teachings of specialists, who do not merely rely on memory, which is not reliable for the science of medicine, but who have a thorough grasp of the system in its entirety—not just piecemeal knowledge. The research of such experts provides a tested repository of direct knowledge of the possible causes and symptoms of every type of disease. The testimony of the patient also constitutes authoritative knowledge.

Clinical diagnosis involves a threefold examination of (1) the patient; (2) the disease; and (3) the medications.

The patient is administered an eightfold test by investigation of: (1) pulse; (2) urine; (3) stool; (4) tongue; (5) voice; (6) touch (skin); (7) eyes; and (8) general features. We mut pass over the details of each test. The physical exam is supplemented by interrogation *(praśna parīkṣa)*. It has a general aspect in which the patient specifies the main complaint and the length of time it has bothered him or her. The physican inquires into the history of the present problem, the history of past illnesses, and the health history of the entire family. Interrogation also covers the personal history of the patient and the environment in which the patient lives. The physician is interested in the patient's living conditions and the health status of his environs. He must know the patient's constitution, likes and dislikes, food habits, addictions, and so on.

The disease is tested through five steps, called *pancha nidāna*, with special reference to (1) the *doṣas*; (2) the *dhātus*; (3) the *malas*; (4) the *srotas*; and (5) the *agnis*.

The first step to get to the precise nature of the disease is to identify the causative factors *(nidāna)*, drawing on a knowledge of the causes of all diseases.

The second step is to look for premonitory symptoms *(pūrvarūpa)*. It is important for the physician to catch the early symptoms of the disease, however undefined, because they assist in diagnosing the disease before it fully develops.

The third step is to notice signs and symptoms *(rūpa)* of the full-blown disease. The symptomatic manifestations of each disease are clearly identified. The *rūpas* are important, because they mark the state of the disease, of the *doṣas, dhātus, agnis,* and *srotas*; they provide the prognosis of the disease; and they suggest the therapies, diet, and regimen that are to be applied.

The fourth step is exploratory *(upashaya)*. Sometimes the findings of the first three steps are not conclusive. This calls for additional exploratory studies to arrive at the actual nature of the disease.

The fifth step is pathogenesis *(samprapti)*. It is the process through which a disease is manifest. Vaidya Shriram Sharma explains: "Diseases are of two types, viz., exogenous and endogenous. If the body vitality is not able to overcome the effects of the causative factors, then endogenous types of diseases occur. These causative factors may either aggravate the *doshas* or suppress the activities of *agnis* or enzymes, leading to *ama* formation. Often both of them occur, simultaneously. This *ama* obstructs the channels of circulation. Thus the nourishment to the tissue cells is reduced, which results in the impairment of the functions of the tissues involved and disease is formed."[164]

Following the examination of the patient and the disease, the third requirement is to select the right medication for whatever ails the patient. The selection is done with attention to the following factors: (1) *doṣas;* (2) *dhātus;* (3) *prakṛti*; (4) nature of the disease; (5) and the organ or system that is directly causative of the problem. In administering the medicine, qualifying factors are taken into account, such as age, season, and so on.

The *tridoṣa* theory, which is central to Āyurveda's understanding of health and disease, is also the basis of treatment. Therefore medicines of antagonistic qualities are selected to correct the disequilibrium. Ayurvedic medications have no side effects. Sharma emphatically points out that "the course of treatment which cures the disease, but produces some other kind of complication, is not a correct line of treatment. Correct treatment cures a disease, without provoking another."[165] The classic form of Āyurveda treatment is the fivefold purification therapy known as *pañcakarma*. These therapies are both curative and preventive. They are used in tandem with therapies that promote longevity *(rasāyana)*.

CHAPTER 3

A HINDU BIOETHICAL ANALYSIS *of Health/Disease and Physician/Patient Relationships in American Society*

HEALTH AND DISEASE

Since the founding of the colonies, Americans have evinced extraordinary fascination for and experimentation with matters of health and disease, and the driving impulse of this interest has been their understanding of the role of religion in the common life. This is abundantly clear when one investigates the major involvements of churches in the building of hospitals, clinics, medical missions, and in their concern for diet, exercise, hygiene, and abstinence from alchohol and drugs. For instance, in 1840 Unitarian minister William Ellery Channing expressed religious sentiments of his times when he articulated his doctrine of health in his lecture on "The Elevation of Laboring Classes." He declared: "Health is the working man's fortune and he ought to watch over it more than the capitalist over his largest investments. Health lightens the efforts of the body and mind."[1] With similar conviction for the church's involvement in health issues, Mary Baker Eddy and the Christian Scientists made the mind-body connection central to their theology, while Mormons, Seventh Day Adventists, Jehovah's Witnesses, and Methodists emphasised lifestyle. Most churches were in the vanguard of the temperance movement. Their common inspiration was Christ as the Great Physician, and Paul's dictum to treat the body as the temple of the Holy Spirit.

In recent years, the religious roots of America's preoccupation with health and disease have been strengthened and surpassed by another penchant of Americans—their fascination for technology to exorcise the demons of disease, debility, and death. As medical practice moved from caring to curing, technology has rapidly become the modus operandi of healthcare delivery, featured by lasers, heart-lung machines, neonatal units, CAT scanners, and genetic engineering. All of this has come with a big financial price that Americans have not been reluctant to pay, even when it has amounted to more than 11 percent of the gross national product. Ethicist Arthur L. Caplan notes that "we spend more than any other nation on the planet for health care and health related services."[2]

Caplan thinks that important political and social values, characteristic of American society, are additionally responsible for our placing a special premium on health and the avoidance of disease. He observes:

> Ours is a highly individualistic society deeply committed to freedom and autonomy as the core values of both our law and morality. Sickness and disease are more threatening to our sense of selfhood and self-assurance than they might be in societies less committed to individualism and less worried about using personal achievement as the measure of a person's worth.[3]

The special meaning of health and disease for American society calls for a clear understanding of the nature of the relationship between health and disease. "Defining what does or does not constitute a disease determines both the authority and power of those charged with alleviating its consequences as well as the scope of the social obligations of those beset by medical problems."[4] Therefore in order to delineate the specific bounds of medicine and the healing arts, we must first construct a precise understanding of these views.

Four major views concerning the relationship between health and disease contend for position. They are:

1. A Value-free Definition of Health
2. A Statistical Conception of Health
3. Health as the Absence of Disease
4. The Normativist View of Health

In each case we will give a brief sketch of the Western position as cited by Caplan and others, and then suggest how insights from Āyurveda can further illuminate more ample definitions of health and disease.

A Value-free Definition of Health and Disease

The first view is based on biological evolution. Its orientation is scientific, basing its understanding of health and disease on empirical facts. As such, it finds no reason to invoke values or morals into its analysis of health. It is confident that we can arrive at objective notions of health or disease without reliance on values. A prominent exponent of this position is philosopher Christopher Boorse. He makes his case in an article "On the Distinction Between Disease and Illness."[5] Boorse claims that inasmuch as all organisms, including humans, are the products of a long course of biological evolution, driven by the demands of survival and reproduction, health is therefore the functioning of any organism in conformity with its natural design, as determined by natural selection. For example, since the organs of our body have evolved in response to natural selection to perform specific functions, a person is healthy to the extent that each organ functions according to its purpose. A state of health exists when a kidney does what it is supposed to do, namely, remove impurities from the body. A state of disease exists when the heart fails to pump blood to organs and tissues. The kidney was designed to eliminate toxins, and the heart to circulate the blood, and a person possessing such organs that accomplish their purposes is said to have a healthy set of kidneys or a strong heart.

In broad terms, Boorse identifies two goals of evolution: survival and reproduction. In order to survive, all organisms have had to learn to adapt. Organisms in which the adaptive traits for reproduction and survival were missing perished from the planet.

As a consequence of "the interaction of genes, phenotypes and environments over time, organisms evolved certain advantageous traits in the struggle for existence. Disease develops whenever there is any impairment of the functions typical of a particular biological species; functions required to achieve the natural goals set by the twin demands of survival and reproduction."[6]

Caplan suspects that on the surface Boorse's analysis may appear "to smuggle in premises or assumptions about values into the analysis of the meanings of health and disease." He hints that the notions of "survival and reproduction" may themselves be "value-laden," and points out that "neither of these terms are used in his analysis in any moralistic or evaluative sense."[7]

Āyurveda is sympathetic to Boorse's borrowings from empirical science, especially his insights from evolution. Unlike some Christian systems of bioethics that are opposed to evolutionary theories, Hindu bioethics is based on the Sāṁkhya system of philosophy that has its own theory of evolution *(pariṇāma-vāda)*, and therefore has a common starting point.

Its basic critique is that Boorse's idea of evolution is not evolved enough. The theory arbitrarily stops at a naturalistic point of development. By contrast, Sāṁkhya explains the origin of the objective universe in all of its infinite diversity, as having evolved from *Prakṛti,* the principle of nature. Since *Prakṛti* is viewed as ultimate and independent, Sāṁkhya's theory of evolution would appear to be naturalistic. However, Sāṁkhya does not stop at this point. It postulates a second entity called *Puruṣa*, the principle of spirit, by means of which we become aware of the physical world in the first place. Thus, while Sāṁkhya attributes an ultimate and independent status to *Prakṛti,* it is more than a philosophy of nature. It postulates the existence of *Puruṣa* on the grounds that objects point to the subject, and that the nonsentient presupposes the sentient. It also argues on the basis of design exhibited by the physical world. To take a medical example, the human body with its myriads of parts points to a purpose for which the body is intended. This teleology, implicit in the microcosm, is similarly manifest in numerous facets of the macrocosm. Sāṁkya reasons, the *telos*, which all these adaptations are designed to serve, is *Puruṣa*. In short, spirit is the principle for which nature evolves.

This declares that the purpose of health in Āyurveda is more than survival and reproduction. When people are hungry and without shelter, they will live only for survival. But once they have survived, other needs come to the fore, which may have nothing to do with survival. These needs express themselves as values. They are not subjective whims, but are the moral articulations of our potencies, and carry an inner authority. Their presence points to the fact that humans can live simultaneously on many levels—physical, mental, or spiritual. Similarly, while reproduction is a legitimate end, for the person who has gotten in touch with his or her spiritual needs, procreation may give way to self-creation. This accounts for the popularity of the celibate ideal among India's holy persons. All these ideals and values do not exist in some mental or spiritual ghetto, but penetrate the deep textures of our body and mind. Therefore it appears medically unsound to think it is possible to have an objective definition of health or disease that does not rely on values. Such a possibility makes nonsense of all our talk about "the quality of life." When a person feels that life has lost its quality, even though all the person's organs are fully functioning, he or she may feel there is little value in mere survival, and this very loss of the will to live has the physiological power to end that life. The truth is: values are vital for health and disease.

The Statistical Concept of Health and Disease

The contention of Boorse that we need not have recourse to any discussions of values or morals in order to identify, understand, or analyze the notions of health and disease is reflected in one of the most common views of health among American physicians. It is the notion that health is a state of normalcy, and disease a state of abnormalcy. The canon by which these judgments are made is not moral but statistical. The midpoint of a spectrum is classified as normal and healthy, whereas the tangents are termed abnormal and unhealthy. In the case when a person's blood pressure or body weight extends beyond the statistical mean, the individual is considered diseased, regardless of whether he or she is experiencing pain or debility.

One social fallout of this statistical approach to health and disease is that the American public is confused by changing trends with respect to the latest figures on what is normal. There are constant shifts regarding what is "in" and "out" in matters of diet (eggs, fish oils, meats), drinks (coffee, tea, wine, beer), operations (tonsil, prostate, circumcision, hysterectomy, breasts), cholesterol, height, weight, vitamins, and so on. Much money is spent and more anxiety is endured by a public that is constantly bombarded by some new study that pontificates on what is "normal" and "abnormal." The situation is bad enough in terms of medical fads that come and go, but it is worse when a patient's doctors prescribe differently. Hence, the growing need for second opinions—which inflate healthcare bills.

Additionally, what is defined as "functional normality" is not always healthful. Janzen points to communities in Africa that have learned to live with certain diseases as constant companions, such as yaws, malaria, intestinal parasites. The trouble is that when habitual conditions are treated as normal, they tend to become justifications for inaction by health care workers and government officials.[8]

For its part, Āyurveda is cautious of all ideas of statistical normalcy to the extent that they fail to give primacy to the particular constitution of the individual. *In Āyurveda, 'normal' and 'abnormal' are not general but specific measurements* that fully take into account the total makeup of the person. This entails a person's anatomy, biochemistry, age, gender, genetics, and environment. For instance, until recently it was common practice for physicians to treat women on the basis of male statistical data, until they discovered there are wide gender variations. Heart disease in men and women does not run a parallel course. Again the amount of alchohol a man can consume before reaching nirvana differs markedly for women. Today we are wiser: 'normal' has gender-specific meanings. The same applies to other categories of comparison. Therefore it is imprecise for physicians to equate factors that depart from the mean as necessarily indicative of disease, especially in the absence of dysfunction or pain.

On the positive side, Āyurveda considers the statistical approach to the definition of health and disease a useful tool for arriving at rough approximations. Its merits in assessing the health status of plants and animals are not in question; but humans must be reckoned with as creatures who belong to a higher rung of the evolutionary ladder and whose lives cannot be reduced to simple empirical facts.

Health as the Absence of Disease

A definition of health that seems to have the least number of complications is that it is the absence of disease. The person in the street will say that she is in good health if she is not experiencing any aches or pains. Similarly, physicians will ask about the health of a person with the question: "Are you having any problems?"

The view of health as the absence of disease is now being critically examined. Clearly health is a matter of degrees. Āyurveda has always been aware of these gradations in health, by distinguishing between healing therapies and promotive therapeutics, as in the case of *rasāyana* therapy, and by distinguishing between diseases that are curable and incurable.

Historically, the notion of health as the absence of disease is rooted in Western classical antiquity, and became popular in the latter part of the nineteenth century with "the discovery of the bacterial causes of the major contagious diseases and of related techniques for their elimination."[9]

In recent years this view has been perpetuated by a reliance on the hope of finding "a magic bullet" that will forever end such scourges as malaria, smallpox, cholera, tuberculosis, and typhus, among others. For a while it was thought that the battle against some of these diseases, such as tuberculosis, was won, but in the past few years these diseases have been making a comeback.

Āyurveda takes umbrage at the notion of health as the absence of disease on two main counts. First it is a negative concept, whereas health in

Āyurveda is a positive, dynamic state that involves the whole person, as well as the environment. Second, as Janzen remarks, it obscures some of "the socioeconomic factors that precipitate or exacerbate these contagious diseases."[10] Āyurveda's preventive stance agrees that if some of the socioeconomic conditions were rectified, there would be less need to rely upon discovery of a "magic bullet" to wipe out diseases. This involves giving as much aid to public health and disease prevention as to pharmaceutical research.

The Normativist View of Health and Disease

Normativists are critics of the view propounded by Christopher Boorse that health and disease can be adequately defined without reference to values.

> Normativists believe that health and disease are concepts that are inherently value-laden. They believe that to understand exactly what it is that these concepts mean or refer to, it is necessary to realize that decisions have to be made about states of the body or mind that must involve considerations of what is desirable or undesirable, useful or useless, good or bad. Normativists argue that no matter how many descriptive facts are known about the body or about the functions of a particular cell or organ system, it is impossible to decide whether or not a particular state of affairs represents health or disease without some reference to a standard or criterion that contains explicit or implicit reference to values.[11]

From the inception of Christianity, disease was defined in metaphysical terms as the work of the divine, the demonic, or the magical. During the early Middle Ages (500–1050), the conversion of Western Europe depended on subduing one manifestation of the supernatural by another. To win the religious following of the pagans, Christian missionaries had to convince them that the Church's power to aid them was greater than that of their pantheistic gods, and that the most effective instruments of the miraculous were invocations of the saints and veneration of their holy relics. The most revered place of this cult of saints and relics was the shrine of Saint Martin at Tours, "where every day we see the blind receive their sight, the deaf their hearing, and the dumb their speech."[12] This brand of spiritual thinking, which focused on the metaphysical etiology of disease and not on whether values played any role in the definition of disease, was laid to rest in academic and medical circles as a result of the mechanical philosophies of Descartes, Boyle, Galileo, and Newton. A trend was thus begun to establish value-free notions of health and disease that conformed to the materialistic approach of scientific medicine.

Today the situation among thinkers is quite different from the views begun in the sixteenth and seventeenth centuries. On the one hand they oppose the materialistic trappings of modern medicine; on the other they do not wish to return to the prescientific outlooks of the Middle Ages. They simply affirm that values form an irreducibe element in the definition of disease, despite modern medicine's commitment to materialism.

The current situation in the West is reminiscent of the historical progression of Āyurveda. The roots of Indian medicine lie in an ancient value-laden ethos, informed by health and disease as the machinations of gods, devils, and sorcerers. Classical Indian medicine succeeded in distancing itself from its magical beginnings and established itself on rational foundations. However, the comparison between East and West ends here. Indian medicine has not found it necessary to forsake the place of values in its understanding of health and disease. To the contrary, its psychosomatic approach domonstrates the interaction between the emotional and physical realms. Hindu bioethics proceeds from a scientific orientation in which matters such as hygiene and good conduct are synthesized. Caraka even goes beyond the psychosomatic analysis of health and disease and includes a third factor: the spirit *(ātman)*. He claims when a person lives in a higher state of consciousness *(prajñā)*, he is ensured health and happiness, whereas when he occupies lower states he becomes prey to disorders, due to intellectual errors *(prajñāparadha)*.

The names of Charles Culver and Bernard Gert stand out among contemporary normativist proponents. They argue that "the core meaning of disease involves the recognition that something is wrong with a person"; that "diseases are actually a subcategory of a more general category" called maladies, such as diseases, injuries, disabilities, and death; and that "what is common to all these conditions is that human beings universally view them as evils."[13]

Indian medicine finds the subjective factor too prominent in the normativist definition of disease, articulated by Culver and Gert. They claim that a condition is called a disease only when members of a society disvalue it as an evil; but a more objective reading of the matter would suggest that a disease could be present, regardless of its recognition. As is pointed out, "Those with hypertension may not feel any loss of capacity but the physician operating with a nonnormative sense of proper physiological functioning can say that disease is present even if the patient would not."[14] Similarly, a nonliterate society may not recognize the presence of dyslexia in one of its children, but a psychologist could detect that an abnormal condition exists.

Indian medicine is disposed toward a normativist stance, but it insists that values be correlated with objective facts. It would go even further and claim that physiological malfunctioning could very well be due to a perversion of values on the part of the individual who suffers from some disease.

Hindu bioethics would also argue that materialistic opponents of the normativist position, who claim on 'scientific grounds' that their own definitions of health and disease are value-free, are often not so free, after all. Consciously or unconsciously, doctors allow their own values to impinge upon their understanding of health in theory and practice. Caplan shows how this happens in the fields of mental health and mental illness. He notes: "A cursory glance of the nineteenth century American medical texts reveals that physicians asserted with all the authority at their disposal that women who enjoyed sexual intercourse or engaged in masturbation were currently afflicted with various forms of mental illness and, in all likelihood, a variety of corresponding physical ailments as well."[15] This highlights the fact that so much "scientific" medicine is actually the practice of a culturally conditioned form of medicine, and the real danger is that the doctors are oblivious of their own biases, and succeed to pass them on to their suggestive patients.

THE PHYSICIAN/PATIENT RELATIONSHIP

The importance of the physician /patient relationship lies in the fact that it is a microcosm of medical ethics as a whole. Currently the subject is under public and governmental scrutiny, because of instances in which physicians failed to treat their patients with due diligence as a result of pressures from their HMOs to curtail services for fiscal reasons. As rewards for their compliance, physicians are given handsome bonuses.

Robert Veatch draws up four models for ethical medicine:

1. The Priestly Model
2. The Engineering Model
3. The Collegial Model
4. The Contractual Model[16]

We will weigh the merits of each model with reference to Āyurvedic principles, which we shall then employ to construct a new entry: 5. The Participatory Model.

The Priestly Model

Robert N. Wilson, sociologist of medicine, sees the physician/patient relationship as having religious overtones. The clinic has "the aura of a sanctuary," in which "the patient must view his doctor in a manner far removed from the prosaic and the mundane."[17] The ethical principle that hallows this tradition is: "Benefit and do no harm to the patient."

The priestly model is grounded in the ancient tradition of paternalism. It is best articulated in the Hippocratic work *Epidemics:* "As to disease, make a habit of two things—to help, or at least to do no harm."[18] The underlying image of paternalism, as the name suggests, is that of the parent-child relationship. The analogy with the *pater* assumes two aspects of the parent's role: "that the father acts beneficently (that is, in accordance with his conception of the interests of his children) and that he makes all or at least some of the decisions relating to his children's welfare, rather than letting them make those decisions. In health care relationships, the analogy is extended further: A professional has superior training, knowledge, and insight and is in an authoritative position to determine the patient's best interests. From this perspective, a health care professional is like a loving parent with dependent and often ignorant and fearful children."[19] Paternalism in the practice of medicine may therefore be defined as the intentional setting aside of a patient's known preferences by a health care professional, in which instance the latter justifies his or her actions by the goal of benefiting or avoiding harm to the patient whose will is superseded. Essentially, the center of decision making is shifted from the patient and is placed in the hands of the professional, who assumes the role of a loving and wise parent.

Since the 1960s, voices have been raised in behalf of the patient's right to make autonomous decisions about his or her medical situation. This has given rise to a focal dilemma in biomedical ethics: Should a patient's autonomy prevail over professional beneficence? Proponents of autonomy claim that a patient's rights in terms of consent, disclosure, confidentiality, and privacy are only sufficiently safeguarded on the basis of the principle of autonomy.

For its part, Hindu bioethics agrees with the contention of Pellegrino and Thomasma that "both autonomy and paternalism are superseded by the obligation to act beneficently. . . . In the real world of clinical medicine, there are no absolute moral principles except the injunction to act in the patient's interest." They provide instances in which a patient's autonomy must be superseded by the physician's beneficence as in the case when a patient irresponsibly rejects lifesaving pencillin treatment for penumococcal or meningococcal meningitis.[22]

Hindu bioethics is opposed to all absolutistic thinking, especially in the context of clinical medicine. It does not believe that medical practice lends itself to making clear-cut choices as to which principle, autonomy or beneficence, is to prevail in any given situation. Instead, Hindu bioethics combines the concerns of the two principles by making beneficence the primary goal in the doctor/patient relationship and respect for the patient's autonomy as a means for setting limits on the doctor's role in pursuit of this task. At all times a doctor is obligated to seek the good of the patient, while avoiding harm, but throughout the process the indiviual's freedom must be protected.

What must the doctor do when the act of telling the truth, in conformity with the patient's right to full disclosure, portends a threat to the patient's very life? Caraka's answer is as follows: "The physician, though observing the signs of death, should not disclose the approaching death without having been requested for. Even on request, he should not express it if it is liable to cause patient's death, or affliction to somebody else."[21] We take this injunction to mean that in the physician's effort to act beneficently and to do no harm in the *extreme case* where death is imminent, the *vaidya* starts off by not volunteering information about the grave conditions. Presumably, in less extreme cases, autonomy would be respected and information about the patient's health status would be volunteered, because the patient is recognized as one leg of a therapeutic tripod in which the patient's informed and active participation is sought. But in this extreme case where full disclosure would do more harm than good, the moral course of action for the physician is to keep quiet and hope for the best. Clearly, this *in extremis* case prompts Caraka to tilt in favor of beneficence, but it would be an error to conclude from this that he has pretensions to elevate the physician into some sort of new priest. In Hindu bioethics the *vaidya* is no priest before whose superior knowledge the patient must morally prostrate. The patient is an equal, endowed with dignity and autonomy to make personal decisions.

The Engineering Model

A consequence of the biological revolution is that it has made physicians scientific, so that in medical practice they function as applied scientists. Their ideal is to be value-free and to base all considerations on 'facts.' The complicity of Nazi doctors in medical atrocities has not shaken this faith in being pure scientists. Veatch points out the folly of this stance, because it is illogical for the scientist and more so the applied scientist to think he or she can be value-free. "Choices must be made daily—in research design, in significant levels of statistical tests, and in perception of the 'significant' observations from an infinite perceptual field, and each of these choices requires a frame of values on which it is based." The argument becomes stronger in reference to an applied field like medicine in which decisions are all the time being made on the basis of what is deemed 'valuable.' "The physician who thinks he can just present all the facts and let the patient make the choices is fooling himself even if it is morally sound and responsible to do this at all the critical points where decisive choices are to be made." In addition, even if it were logically possible for the physician to divest his or her practice of all value considerations, it would be morally catastrophic to do so. "It would make him an engineer, a plumber making repairs, connecting tubes and flushing out clogged systems, with no questions asked."[23]

For Hindu bioethics, the physician cannot be reduced to a plumber, because a physician is expected to function at all times as a professional invested with moral integrity. Further, the physician is a significant leg of the tripod, having something special to offer in terms of professional knowledge and skill, and hence it is not fitting for the patient to assume full control and for the doctor simply to engineer and expedite his or her wishes.

The Collegial Model

Veatch explains that the collegeal model is built on the twin values of trust and confidence that are justified when there is mutual commitment to shared goals. The collegial model not only makes for the most harmonious form of human interaction; it ensures "an equality of dignity and respect, an equality of value contributions" missing in other models.

Hindu bioethics welcomes the collegial pursuit of the common goal of ending illness and preserving the health of the patient, but it stops short of the notion that the patient is the physician's "pal." Even if this association were possible, it would not be desirable, because, though acting in concert, the roles of the physician and of the patient are distinctly different. The legs of the "tripod" are equal though separate.

In addition, Hindu bioethics is gently amused by the assumption of the collegial model of "mutual loyalty and goals, of common interest," given the social realities of ethnic, class, economic, and value differences that prevail. Veatch shares this skepticism and considers the assumption of common interests that are necessary for the collegial model to succeed "a mere pipedream."[24] By comparison, the stance of Hindu bioethics is more provisional, insisting only on the need to ensure equality in the area of moral significance between doctor and patient; anything more would be creating the utopian assumption of collegiality.

4. *The Contractual Model*

Veatch envisions the contractual model along the lines of a marriage "contract" in which two persons interact with one another in terms of obligations and expected benefits for the couple. He spells out the relationship thus:

> With the contractual relationship there is a sharing in which the physician recognizes that the patient must maintain freedom of control over his own life and destiny when significant choices are to be made. Should the physician not be able to live with his conscience under those terms the contract is not made or is broken. This means that there will have to be relatively greater open discussion of the moral premises hiding in medical decisions before and as they are made.
>
> With the contractual model there is a sharing in which the patient has legitimate grounds for trusting that once the basic value framework for medical decision making is established on the basis of the patient's own values, the myriads of minute medical decisions which must be made day in and day out in the care of the patient will be made by the physician within the frame of reference.

Thus the contractual model allows for "realistic sharing" in the decision-making process by the patient and physician, without either feeling any diminution of their "moral integrity." It assures patient control of decision making in the individual level "without the necessity of insisting that the patient participate in every trivial decision."[25]

On the credit side of the ledger, Hindu bioethics salutes the contractual model's affirmation of the basic norms of freedom, dignity, truth telling, promise keeping, and justice, as well as its premises of trust and confidence. Compared with the other models, only the contractual model makes it possible to have a true sharing of ethical authority and responsibility.

On the debit side, Hindu bioethics holds back its full support for the contractual model on the following counts shared by several prominent ethicists, such as Daniel Callahan, C. Fried, J. Ladd, R. D. Masters, and M. Siegler. Howard Brody neatly summarizes these charges, which we give below in paraphrase.

It is a misrepresentation to say that a patient and physician begin their relationship with some sort of cut-and-dried contract. A good part of the relationship rests on understanding that is not explicitly articulated. There is a deep ethical content to the relationship, which the contractual model overlooks because of the prominence it gives to financial aspects. Similarly, ethical notions such as duties and goals are overlooked in favor of concentration upon narrow legal rights, and this tends to make the contractual model legalistic. It raises the specter of medical ethics being replaced by medical law. Legalistic reasoning elevates patient autonomy, but this should not incur oversight of the moral principles of patient benefit and avoidance of harm. Finally, Brody charges that contractual models create a medical culture of minimalist thinking. "Instead of asking, 'How may I cultivate and nourish this relationship over the long term for better service to the patient's welfare?,' the models encourage the physician to ask, 'What's the least I can get away with in the short run without violating any explicit rights of the patient.'"[26]

The Participatory Model

Whereas in the patriarchal model the physician is viewed as a priest who exercises so much moral authority that the freedom and dignity of the patient are eclipsed; and whereas in the engineering model the patient is in full control, while the doctor is denuded of his own ethical judgments; and whereas in the collegial model physician and patient pose as pals; and whereas in the contractual model the emphasis is more on financial and legal aspects and less on social and ethical aspects; the *participatory model* recognizes elements of truth in each model, based on a view of the *patient as person*, who is both *dependent and responsible*, and therefore in equal need of *beneficence and autonomy*. In such an existential association, neither the doctor nor patient is accorded a role of primacy, but both are expected to work as a team, meeting each new situation as it arises. A distinguishing mark of this understanding of the doctor/patient relationship is that it is *not streamlined*, like the others; the reason being that it declines to make any one principle absolute.

The centerpiece of the participatory model is Caraka's paradigm of "four-legged therapeutics."[27] Reference has already been made to this theme, but we repeat its main outlines here. Elsewhere the relationship is described in terms of a tripod.

As propounded by Lord Ātreya: "Physician, drug, attendant and patient, this is the quadruple which, if endowed with qualities, leads to alleviation of disorders."[28] Disorders refer to the disequilibrium of the *dhātus*, which produce unhappiness, while health is equilibrium and happiness. Health, being the normal state of the person, is the good that must be sought by all means. The heart of therapeutics is the employment of the strengths of the total quadruple ("excellent four") in order to reestablish equilibrium.

The excellent qualities of each participant are then repeated.[29]

Physician. "Excellence in theoretical knowledge, extensive practical experiences, dexterity and cleanliness—this is the quadruple of qualities of a physician."

Drug. "Abundance, effectivity, various pharmaceutical forms and normal composition—these are the four qualities of drugs."

Attendant. "Knowledge of attendance, dexterity, loyalty and cleanliness—these are four qualities of an attendant."

Patient. "Memory, obedience, fearlessness and providing all information about the disorder—these are the qualities of a patient."[30]

Thus, the participatory aspect of the doctor/patient relationship is affirmed by likening it to a four-legged table in which each leg is "endowed with qualities" which lead to "alleviation of disorders." If any one leg is removed or diminished, the whole table falls. The arrangement is clearly one of *complementarity among equals*.

For his part, the patient contributes to his healing and health by carefully monitoring himself and keeping tabs on all developments. He must entertain no negative emotions, while he maintains faith in his doctor, keeps the doctor fully informed, and follows directions. Because of the prominence given to clinical diagnosis, the physician depended heavily on the patient for accurate feedback. The physician was to keep record of the signs, symptoms, stages of the disease, condition of the patient's *doṣas, dhātus, agnis, and malas*, among several other particulars in respect to food, time, place, exercise, lifestyle, and family history. Pregnant women had special responsibilites for monitoring the days from conception till parturition.

At the same time the eminence of the physician is left in no doubt. The physician's high importance is based, not on professional status, but on competence and character. He must be schooled in medical theory and practice, devoted to learning and rationality, and always ready to act. In character he must be compassionate and friendly toward his patient, and make the patient the focus of his practice. Upon his initiation, the young doctor is told: "When you join the medical profession and wish success in work, earnings of wealth, fame, and heaven after death, you should always think of the welfare of all living beings. . . . You should make effort to provide health to the patients by all means. You should not think ill of the patients even at the cost of your life."[31]

Because of his "excellence" in therapeutics, as well as his personal probity, the physician is granted a pivotal role. "As earth, stick, wheel, thread, etc., do not serve the purpose (of making a pitcher) without the potter, the other three legs are in the same position without the physician."[32] The physician as potter has indeed a principal role to play, but the clay and the wheel also have their parts, each according to its own "excellence." The functions are complementary, with no chance of mistaking the "potter" for a "patriarch" or "priest." All pretensions of patriarchalism were warded off by the need for modesty. "Though possessed of knowledge one should not boast. . . . people are offended by boastfulness of even those who are otherwise good and authoritative." Moreover, "there is no limit at all to the Science of Life. . . . The entire world is the teacher to the intelligent . . . knowing this well, thou shouldst listen and act according to the words of instruction of even an unfriendly person."[33] That is, the physician must acknowledge his or her fallibility and be open to accommodating a second opinion.

The doctor/patient relationship also mandated rights of privacy. The physician is instructed: "The peculiar customs of the patient's household shall not be made public."[34] A protective net is thrown over the home the physician enters. In the first place, the doctor's "speech, mind, intellect and senses" should be disciplined to attend only to the patient's needs; not to take inventory of private and personal matters. He is also forbidden to make known to other parties any of the privileged information he has gained from his house call. Such safeguards were set in place to build trust and confidence in the doctor/patient relationship. In a modern setting, *the right of privacy* would mean that the *vaidya* would refuse disclosure of information to employers and insurance companies, when it could be used against the patient in terms of loss of job or of medical coverage.

The doctor/patient relationship was also governed by rules of disclosure. Reference has been made to the text: "Even knowing that the patient's span of life has come to its close, it shall not be mentioned by thee there, where if so done, it would cause shock to the patient or to others."[35] In addition to what was said in our discussion of the patriarchal model, we must point out that the cultural setting of this injunction is important, wherein the physician and the family members are closely united, without being "pals." The question of disclosure is treated circumstantially: where it is obvious that the bad news will make things worse, it is *prudent* not to traumatize the patient or loved ones. Where, however, the news is not expected to produce a shock, there is no policy against full disclosure. On the face of it this sounds like crypto paternalism. Beneficence is being elevated at the expense of autonomy. The *vaidya* is acting like a priest in disguise. Actually, the premises for limited disclosure were the *vaidya*'s (1) intimate knowledge of his patient, based on past responses; (2) familiarity with the *family*; and (3) knowledge of the stage of the disease.

How well would Caraka's rules of disclosure stack up in a modern setting?

First we must reckon with legal aspects of the issue. In an American city such as Honolulu, the law is clear. All risks and benefits must be explained, including the alternative of no treatment at all. It is legally incumbent on physicians to tell patients everything. If a doctor does not, it is negligence. Hawaii law in particular requires a physician to explain fully the consequences of treatment, including any long- or short-term risks, side effects, and alternative treatments. The law recognizes the patient's autonomy and freedom to make his or her own choices.

In the context of standard therapy, Hawaii's law is not in conflict with Caraka's dictum that doctors may withold information from the patient if it *injuriously affects* the patient's health of mind and body. However, that doctrine cannot be invoked when a patient faces a heart transplant or other nontraditional therapy.

The bottom line of this issue of truth telling is that there is no medical way of really knowing when life is worth living. Only a patient can decide if life is worth living. Perhaps those feelings of worth are the only things that keep the patient going. But should a doctor, in the interests of mechancically telling the truth, say "You have a 50 per cent chance of survival," "There is no cure," that doctor may be *close to the facts*, but his patient may be *closer to his grave*.

Focus on the *vaidya's* relationship with the individual patient did not overlook the social dimensions of the doctor's duties. "No persons, who are hated by the king or who are haters of the king or who are hated by the public or who are haters of the public, shall receive treatment. Similarly, those who are extremely abnormal, wicked, and of miserable character and conduct, those who have not vindicated their honor, those who are on the point of death, and similarly women who are unattended by their husbands or guardians shall not receive treatment."[36] The physican, under license by the state, was obliged to observe all the social sanctions against such persons, presumably for the greater good.

CONCLUSION

What are the implications for today of Caraka's formulation of the doctor/patient relationship conceived as a stool having four legs?

On the plus side, the technical quality of medical care administered by the modern physician is simply unmatched. He or she works with other specialists in a team, using such innovations as imaging techniques to diagnose illnesses and laser technology to repair them. In all the surveys, patients give their physicians high marks for such competence and expertise.

On the minus side, the same patients complain that in the diagnosis of their physical and psychological problems, physicians do not give them the opportunity to talk, to be listened to, to have the chance to say what really ails them, and to have their emotional concerns properly addressed. The communication style of the physician is often technical, information-oriented, controlling, and physician-centred. The doctor seems to have a preconceived notion of what is wrong with the person, and employs yes and no answers only to confirm preset hunches.

Communication problems not only surface on the *diagnostic* level but on the level of *instruction*. The inscrutable hieroglyphics of doctors is matched by their mysterious explanations, wrapped in foreign phrases. Doctors tend to overrate their communication skills, and underrate the patient's ability to grasp complex processes, when explained in plain language. This leaves the patient in a quandary about the facts of his or her illness, causing stress. Ignorance of the facts can carry over into the patient's failure to comply with instructions, not really knowing whether HDL is the good cholesterol or LDL the bad stuff.

Hindu bioethics would consider the communication style of the modern medic as a device derived from *disease-oriented views of health*. The goal of the Western specialist is to connect the patient's complaint with some form of organic pathology, and the most efficient way to do this is for the expert to determine what pieces of information count. This mode of questioning is alien to Āyurveda with its positive view of health, its dependence on all senses for diagnosis, and its understanding of the patient as an individual who cannot be read by the book or with one eye on the clock.

Also, Āyurveda is at the opposite extreme of the "high control style." Being patient-centered, it promotes a style in which patients are questioned in an open-ended manner, with due consideration to individuality, so that the patient can determine what is important to relate. The physician avoids medical jargon, asks for clarification, and encourages joint decision making. In essence, the physician tries to understand the meaning of the illness from the patient's point of view. Nor are emotions played down as superfluous to the illness, because Āyurveda's psychosomatic approach recognizes that a patient's feelings do impact illness, for better or for worse.

The clash of these two powerful cultures, with very different ways of viewing the world, was featured recently in *Time*, entitled "The Science of Yoga" (April 23, 2001). It says: "The Indian tradition develops metaphors and ways of describing the body (life forces, energy centers) as it is experienced from the inside out. The Western tradition looks at the body from the outside in, peeling it back one layer at a time, believing only what it can see, measure and prove in randomized, double-blind tests. The East treats the person; the West treats the disease" (p. 56).

Finally, the participatory role accorded to patients in Āyurveda means that they have to bear much of the responsibility for establishing good rapport, particularly now that managed care has changed the doctor-patient relationship. Patients have to become savvy in communicating with their doctors, because that is one of the few things they can control in today's health care.

PART TWO

ISSUES AT THE BEGINNING AND END OF LIFE

CHAPTER 4

TECHNOLOGY AND THE WOMB

In Part One we sought to present the basic tenets of the Hindu ethical system. In Part Two we attempt to clarify the implications of these fundamental ethical principles for select moral issues that raise new challenges in medical contexts.

In 1987 the Congregation for the Doctrine of the Faith, the Vatican agency that is responsible for monitoring orthodoxy, issued a forty-page document entitled *Instruction on Respect for Human Life in Its Origin and on the Dignity of Procreation: Replies to Certain Questions of the Day*. Though the document is not published as an infallible pronouncement, it does carry definitive authority to this day. Its purpose is to denounce virtually all of the rapidly spreading methods of artificial procreation, deeming them to be violations of both the rights of humans and the laws of God. At a press conference in Rome, head of the congregation, Joseph Cardinal Ratzinger, said: "What is technologically possible is not also morally admissible."[1] The *Instruction* sternly admonishes that a child must never be desired or conceived as the "product of an intervention of medical or biological techniques"—that would be tantamount to reducing the child to "an object of scientific technology."

In addition to its insistence that Catholics submit to its teachings, the document also calls upon governments to enact legislation prohibiting a number of the controversial reproductive techniques. As a result the *Instruction* has provoked widespread debate not only on the ethics of the reproductive techniques it discusses but on the propriety of the Vatican's attempt to influence public policy on a medical issue, particularly in pluralistic societies.

The major practices condemned are:

1. Artificial Insemination
2. In Vitro Fertilization

3. Surrogate Motherhood
4. Embryo Experiments

What is the position of Hindu bioethics in respect to these methods of conception, which remain controversial issues in the West? We focus on methods 2 and 3.

IN VITRO FERTILIZATION AND EMBRYO TRANSFER (IVF-ET)

The procedure in contention is for a woman to undergo hormone treatment to stimulate the follicles to produce eggs. Once the follicles have matured, the physician removes some eggs through the surgical procedure of laparoscopy. The eggs are deposited in a culture medium in a petri dish. Sperms are then added to the eggs for fertilization. After a couple of days, the fertilized embryos are transferred to the woman's womb. Following some bed rest, the embryos implant in the uterus, and from that point onwards, the normal course of pregnancy proceeds.

Hindu bioethics would not find difficulty with IVF-ET in respect to the harm/benefit ratio. To be sure, one must consider the possible harm attendant upon the hormone therapy; the surgical laparoscopy under general anesthesia; the risks incurred by the extra-corporeal management of the egg, sperm, and embryo; the limited rate of success; and the high emotional and financial costs; but all of this must be measured against the wishes and rights of the couple. In addition to the basic human urge to have one's own biological offspring, Hindus are guided by religion in respect to progeny. The Law Books state: "To be mothers were women created, and to be fathers men; religious rites, therefore are ordained in the Veda to be performed (by the husband) together with the wife."[2] Male progeny was especially prized. The epics agree with the rest of the literature: "Let a man wed and beget sons, for in them there is a profit greater than any other profit." The sonless man was born to no end, and he who does not propagate himself is godless *(adharmika)*; for to carry on the blood is the highest duty and virtue.[3] It is therefore logical that in the four stages of life, that of the householder is ranked the highest.

In ordinary cases, Hindu bioethics would want to limit IVF-ET to married couples, using their own gametes in order to maximize the chance of both physical and emotional success for the child. However, there is provision in the Hindu tradition for use of donor sperm. One precedent for this exigency is found in an ancient form of sexual union known as *niyoga*. Its purpose was the impregnation of a wife of an impotent or dead man so that his family may be preserved, and he may have sons to offer oblations for the welfare of his soul in the next world. The custom has Vedic origins, possibly going back to the practice whereby the brother-in-law extends his hand to the wife of the deceased on the funeral pyre. In the Law Books *niyoga* was strictly accepted as a dispassionate duty.

According to Gautama, the oldest Dharma Sūtra writer:

> A woman whose husband is dead and who desires offspring (may bear a son) to her brother-in-law.
>
> Let her obtain the permission of her Gurus, and let her have intercourse during the proper season only.[4]
>
> Only two children are permitted through this arrangement.

If more than two children are born, and if no prior conditions have been set, the offspring belong equally to the husband of the woman and to the begetter. "But being reared by the husband (it belongs to him.)"[5]

Manu does not approve of the custom of *niyoga*, but acknowledges its social reality, and circumscribes it with strict rules. He says:

> On failure of issue (by her husband) a woman who has been authorised, may obtain (in the) proper (manner prescribed), the desired offspring by (cohabitation with) a brother-in-law or (with some other) *Sapiṇḍa* (of her husband).
>
> He (who is) appointed to (cohabit with) the widow shall (approach her) at night anointed with clarified butter and silent (and) beget one son, by no means a second.[6]

Manu does concede that under circumstances a second son may be lawfully procreated, but is adamant that the subsequent relationship between the begetter and the widow be strctly formal.

In addition to cases in which the husband has died, sterile or impotent men could, as last resort, appoint a close relative, usually a brother, to produce offspring on their behalf. The epics are full of stories indicating that holy men were often called upon for this purpose and were able to meet the demands.

The best known instance of *niyoga* is recorded in the Mahābhārata.[7] It is the story of King Pāṇḍu who, on pain of instant death, is cursed not to copulate. Yet he needs sons to perform rituals that will sustain his ethereal body when he dies. Therefore he urges his wife Kuntī to find a proxy with whom she can produce offspring for himself.

Being a woman of probity, Kuntī passionately rejects the request: "Thou must not speak thus to me, who am a virtuous wife, and find my delight by thee, O lotus-eyed one. But thou, O hero, wilt beget with me, in lawful wise, children endowed with heroes' strength. I will go into heaven together with thee. Come thou to me that there may be offspring. I myself, indeed, could draw nigh unto no other man in my thoughts but thee. And what man on earth were more excellent than thou?" Then Kuntī narrates to Pāṇḍu the ancient legend of the loving wife who even conceived children through her dead husband; and ends by saying he will enable her to conceive in a purely spiritual manner, by recourse to the yogic powers he has accumulated by strict asceticism. However, the possibility of resorting to *immaculate conception* did not appeal to King Pāṇḍu. Finally, the wife accedes to her husband's wishes and, through the love proxyship contrived by her husband, produces Yudhiṣṭhira by union with Dharma; Bhīma with the god of wind; and Arjuna with god Indra. Two other sons were begotten by Pāṇḍu's second wife, because, had Kuntī a fourth son by this method, she would have become one that is unbridled *(svairiṇi)*, and with a fifth she would be deemed a worthless woman *(bandhakī)*.

In modern situations, legal questions are raised in respect to the status of the donor of the sperm. Is he to be treated as the 'father' of the offspring he has sired, and what are his rights to the child?

Manu was familiar with such questions even in his times. He presents differing opinions: "They (all) say that the male issue (of a woman) belongs to the lord, but with respect to the (meaning of the term) lord the revealed texts differ; some call the begetter (of the child the lord), others declare (that it is) the owner of the soil."[8] After arguing for the biological importance of the "seed" relative to the "field," Manu resorts to proprietary models to establish legal ownership and rights. "Those who, having no property in a field, but possessing seed-corn, sow it in another's soil, do indeed not receive the grain of the crop which may spring up" (vs. 49). "Thus men who have no marital property in women, but sow their seed in the soil of others, benefit the owner of the woman; but the giver of the seed reaps no advantage" (vs. 51). In terms of the comparative importance of the seed and the womb, "the receptacle is more important than the seed" (vs. 52).

Behind the crude analogies with land and livestock, the principled thinking seems to be that since the proxy is acting in behalf of the woman's husband, and since the wife brings the child to birth, all rights are on the side of the husband who has contracted with the agent for begetting his offspring.

While this was the standard legal procedure, there was room for exceptions whereby the natural father and the husband of the woman could have mutual paternal rights. Manu: "If by a special contract (a field) is made over (to another) for sowing, then the owner of the seed and the owner of the soil are both considered in this world as sharers of the (crop)" (vs. 54).

Of course, this liberal acceptance of sperm donation "in times of misfortune" *(apad)* found little favor with conservatives like Āpastamba, who argued that only the donor benefits from this deal, because the son is biologically his, and only a son born from one's loins was fit to offer oblations for the departed soul.

The conservative position finally prevailed, but by the beginning of the Christian era *niyoga* was roundly disapproved. Medieval literature places it among customs that were once permitted but now denied *(kalivarjya)*. However, the intent was not wasted. We know that the widespread practice of polygamy in early times was elevated to *a religious duty* in the quest for a man to produce a son. Should the husband, and not the wife, be sterile, the man could resort to other methods. Basham notes: "From several stories in the Epics and elsewhere it appears that holy men of special sanctity were often in demand for this purpose, and practice of this kind are said to take place occassionally even at the present day."[9]

It is clear that one reason the practice of sperm donation in the modern West runs into moral and legal problems, in contrast to the ancient Indian practice, is the definition of marriage. In the West, sexual intercourse tends to dominate the relationship, as the be all and end all of marriage. In the Hindu tradition, sexual intercourse is an important facet of the relationship but it is not the only one. Marriage *(vivāha)* and family *(kutumba)* are intrinsically related, their ultimate purpose being the begetting of a son by whom *mokṣa* is attained. It is this end that makes *vivaha* obligatory and justifies all *emergency means* to attain that end, including means that would ordinarily be deemed immoral. The morality of such situations resides in the *intention* and *outcome* of the act (progeny), and not in the act (intercourse) itself.

Thus, whereas the Roman Catholic Church categorically opposes the act of introducing sperm into a womb from a husband, and also sperm from a "third party" donor other than the husband, Hindu bioethics would certainly not be averse to the husband's donated sperm, and could be hospitable to the third-party donation when it is carried out under socially accepted specifications, as was the intent of the ancient custom of *niyoga*.

Furthermore, a major aspect of Rome's opposition to embryo transfer is the employment of technology whereby eggs are fertilized outside the womb in laboratory vessels, and the resulting embryo is then implanted in the womb. Pope Pius XII criticized this in vitro concept as early as 1956. By contrast, as far back as the Mahābhārata, there is a myth, which Desai aptly calls "science-fiction," that describes embryonic development as taking place in pots, "not unlike test tubes."[10]

This is the story of how Gāndhārī, wife of the blind king Dhṛitarāshṭra, was granted a boon for a hundred sons by the sage Vyāsa. Gāndhārī conceived, but was unable to deliver for two years, at which time, fainting with pain, she aborted "a dense ball of clotted blood." Vyasa appeared and ordered that a hundred pots be filled with ghee. He sprinkled water on the ball of flesh, which then proceeded to fragment into a hundred embryos. These were deposited in the pots and closely guarded. In due time, the long awaited hopes of Dhṛitarāshṭra and Gāndhārī were fulfilled with the birth of many offspring.

The Mahābhārata story sheds some light on the ethics of in vitro fertilization. It envisages a technique of last resort for couples who want offspring, and demonstrates remarkable prescience in the possibility of *embryological development outside the female body.* As an Indian physician, Desai, comments:

> A myth like this could be advanced to show the ethical acceptability of test-tube babies for Hindus. Similarly, a case could be made for ovum donation and the implantation of a fertilized ovum. I myself encountered in a clinical situation a couple's attempt to conceive a child by having the wife sleep with the husband's friend. Infertility is a major source of stress, especially for women, who bear the brunt of the social stigma and psychological strife.[11]

SURROGATE MOTHERHOOD

This method involves a woman bearing a child on behalf of others, often for payment, through artificial insemination or the implantation of a fertilized egg. The practice drew national attention in 1987 through publicity of an anguished struggle between two New Jersey couples in the so-called Baby M. case.

Mary Beth Whitehead, a twenty-nine-year-old housewife, agreed to bear a child for William Stern, a biochemist, and his wife, Elizabeth, a forty-one-year-old pediatrician.

Under the contract arranged by the Infertility Center of New York, the couple was to pay Whitehead $10,000 to be artificially inseminated with Stern's sperm. Mrs. Stern planned to adopt the infant.

But after giving birth, Whitehead and her husband changed their minds and refused to turn the child over to the Sterns, triggering a bitter court case. The Stern's attorneys had argued that everyone entered the contract in good faith and that Whitehead reneged. The court in New Jersey upheld the validity of a surrogate mother contract, but the New Jersey Supreme Court reversed the decision.

Legality aside, what is the moral status of surrogate motherhood?

The Roman Catholic Church has condemned surrogate parenthood. Father Richard A. McCormick calls the procedure "specious." His critique focuses on societal risks, involving the loss of such basic values as the institution of marriage, "the notion of parenting, the good of the spouses, the self-identity and overall good of the prospective child, the dignity of women . . . the integrity of the medical profession."[12]

Hindu bioethics shares McCormick's concern for any diminution to family values. It faces squarely the harms and benefits to the couple, the surrogate, and to the child.

Harms

For the couple, surrogacy involves the expenditure of huge fees for legal and medical services. There is also the stress, involving family and friends, of having to defend a procedure that many consider immoral, "weird," unnatural. Besides, surrogates are known to have had sex with husbands/lovers during their fertile period; have not always taken good care of their health; and have been known, as in the case of Mary Beth Whitehead, to be capable of changing their minds, all of which can bring anxiety attacks upon the stress-ridden couple.

Opponents of surrogacy fear it may become an option for women who do not want to interrupt their careers or education with a pregnancy, an argument that was brought up in the New Jersey case.

For the surrogate, there could be much pain and misery connected with the insemination process, pregnancy, and delivery. Her greatest struggle would be with her maternal instincts as she has to hand over the child whom she has carried and to whom she has given birth.

Some have argued that the practice of surrogacy exploits poor women who enter a surrogate contract—usually with well-to-do couples—only because they need money.

For the child there is the risk of psychosocial harm. Surrogate mothering bifurcates genetic and gestational from social parentage. The mother who bears the child does not bring it up. This separation can present difficulties for the child when the facts are known. Were the child interested but unsuccessful in connecting with the absent mother, it could produce feelings of rootlessness, rejection, and ruin of self-esteem. Ethicists (Leon Kass, Paul Ramsey, et al.) correctly point out that "collaborative reproduction" confuses the lineage of children and distorts the meaning of family as we know it in the West.

The most serious source for confusing family lines occurs in the event the couple chooses to cultivate close relations with the surrogate and her husband and children. The child could be at a terrible loss to understand its peculiar relations to these people from another home.

Benefits

Along with the harms, Hindu bioethics also evaluates the benefits that may accrue to the couple, the surrogate, and the child.

Surrogacy meets the needs of an *infertile couple* in a marvelous way: they can have a healthy child who has the genes of one partner. For many, this is more preferable than having to adopt the child of some other couple, with all of the problems attendant upon going through an adoption agency.

The surrogate also stands to benefit. Usually she has had children of her own. As the *natural mother* of the child, we may assume she has feelings of pride for her reproductive role, and is motivated with sufficient feelings of altruism to be able to present an infertile couple with the gift of life. Of course, there must be recompense for her completion of the pregnancy. The fee she receives for her *nine months of labor* can hardly be reduced to a commercial transaction. (Whitehead received $10,000, but did not accept it.) We recall that in Kentucky the state Supreme Court ruled in 1986 that surrogate motherhood was not the same as baby-selling, a practice prohibited in all states.

The child is the chief beneficiary of all, because if it were not for the surrogate arrangement, he or she would not have seen the light of day. In time, questions of identity would surely rise, producing some confusion, but this would be half those of an adopted child, because one parent would be known.

The notion of surrogacy does not startle the Indian mind as it does the theological mind of the West. The reason is that the Indian scriptures, with their fantastic exploits of gods and goddesses, have attuned the popular mind to being open to such possibilities. Desai cites one such story of the birth of Krishṇa and his brother Balarāma, and suggests it "may guide the resolution of modern dilemmas concerning reproduction." He recounts:

> King Kamsa was warned that the eighth child of his sister Devaki and Vasudeva would slay him. The king imprisoned the couple and killed the first six of their children. The seventh was saved by a goddess's intervention: the embryo was removed from the womb of Devaki and implanted in the womb of Vasudeva's other wife. The eighth child, Krishna himself, was saved by an exchange with another newborn who was later killed by the evil king. [13]

In India, such legends are more than mere myths. The division between gods and mortals is not absolute, as we find in semitic religions, and therefore the actions of the gods are looked upon as paradigmatic for humans. The act by which the embryo was implanted in the womb of the surrogate mother and brought to term may be emulated by humans.

On the morality of the payment of fees to the surrogate, the Mahābhārata has instances in which it is considered acceptable that a begetter by proxy be paid. By one account, when King Vicitravīrya had died childless, his half-brother Bhiṣma, who carried on the government, said: "I will also name the means *(hetu)* that is necessary for the propagation and increase of the Bharata blood. Hearken thou unto it from my lips: Some Brahman gifted with excellences must be invited for money to raise up children on Vicitravīrya 's field for him."[14] Often these individuals are Brāhmins, "gifted with excellences," who are invited by some king to raise up children on *his field* for the benefit of his family. It would seem that if it is acceptable that a male be paid, as in this instance, then it is much more morally justifiable that a surrogate mother be monetarily rewarded for her gestational role.

Additionally, a case can be made for the morality of surrogacy within the Indian tradition, on the basis of its past custom of *niyoga* (and related devices). In principle both are the same. Whereas in *niyoga* the proxy supplies the sperm, in surrogacy the woman supplies the uterus. Surrogacy is a case of *reverse niyoga*, though with considerably greater investments on the part of the woman, and hence carrying greater moral weight.

Finally, amid all the questions that are raised in opposition to surrogacy: Is it in fact buying and selling of children? Is it the treatment of the child as a commodity? Is it the exploitation of poor women? For the Indian tradition, all these questions pale in the light of the fact that a childless couple has found a way to satisfy deep human desire to have a child of their own, having weighed all risks and benefits, and having acted in a collaborative manner that is just and legal.

CHAPTER 5

DILEMMAS AT BIRTH

SHOULD EVERY BABY BE SAVED?

A medical revolution in the 1980s that assured the survival of very tiny premature babies has led to a generation of disabled children who are often retarded, handicapped, severely nearsighted, and inattentive. Most of these problems resulted because their bodies were simply too undeveloped to cope with the world outside the womb. These were the findings of a study of the Case Western Reserve University (CWRU) in Cleveland, which investigated babies born between 1982 and 1986.[1]

Their disabilities varied greatly. Some of these children were blind or could not walk; others were virtually normal or had only subtle learning problems.

In general, though, doctors found these youngsters to be at serious disadvantage in every skill required for adequate performance in school.

This is the unfortunate side of a seeming medical miracle.

It is gratifying that modern technology can make 'miracle babies' by keeping them alive in artificial wombs. Before 1975 only 6 percent of babies with birth weights under 2 lbs. 2 ozs. managed to live. By the first half of the 1980s, the survival rate for such children had jumped 48 percent. Those odds continue to improve. Now babies weighing 2 lbs. 30 ozs. to 3 lbs. 5 ozs. have a 90 percent chance of survival. Even so, *often the life for which they have been saved carries a heavy price.*[2]

The cost is both financial and physical, raising many ethical questions.

A study of care for preemies at Stanford University Hospital revealed the average cost was about $160,000. A 1990 report in the *American Journal of Diseases of Children* indicated that $2.6 billion is spent nationally on neonatal intensive care each year.[3] Notwithstanding the high cost for the extraordinary treatments, half the survivors face a lifetime of disabilities cited in the CWRU study.

By federal law U.S. doctors are required to commence treatment of all babies, except hopeless cases. This often develops into an ethical issue, because *the very technology that can save the life of a baby dooms it to profound handicaps down the road.*

In such dilemmatic situations, the Hindu physician first assesses harms and benefits, and selects only those cases that will benefit by treatment. Cases are not that clear, so the physician would err on the side of life and begin treatment immediately on all viable newborns. Through periodic checks, progress is monitored, and where brain damage or the prospects of death are indicated, treatment is stopped. That decision is made after consulting with the parents of the infant.

Some doctors take the position that it is their responsibility not to give a family a handicapped child. Such an attitude is not embraced by Hindu bioethics which considers that *life has its own value, handicapped or not.*

However, the starting point of Āyurveda is to avoid premature births, and the agonizing decisions that follow by providing expectant mothers with adequate prenatal care. This means taking prenatal care programs to poor pregnant women who fail to see doctors and to mothers who use 'crack' or other drugs that induce prematurity. Putting together such programs will have their costs, but they will pay their way, considering the horrendous costs of neonatal intensive-care units. The State of Hawaii has saved thousands of dollars by implementing prenatal care programs.

SHOULD ANIMAL TRANSPLANTS BE GIVEN TO HUMANS?

After twenty-one days of battling to preserve the fragile life of Baby Fae, heart surgeon Dr. Leonard Bailey of Loma Linda University Medical Center in California announced: "Today we grieve the loss of this patient's life. Infants with heart disease yet to be born will some day soon have the opportunity to live, thanks to the courage of this infant and her parents. We are remarkably encouraged by what we have learned from Baby Fae."[4] So ended an extraordinary experiment that had captured the attention of the world and made medical history. For three weeks the 5-lb. infant had survived with the heart of a seven-month-old female baboon.

The heart transplant was necessary because the child was born with a fatal defect called hypoplastic left heart.

Several ethical questions arise from the case of Baby Fae, including the wisdom of the doctors in using an animal heart when a human organ might have been preferable. However, we focus on the ethics of placing a baboon heart into the chest of this human child, inasmuch as it excited enormous indignation among several people. From the pulpits of America, the message sounded forth: only humans are made in the "image of God," and nothing should be done to change that sacred identity. It was strongly felt that the dignity of Baby Fae had been defaced, that some sacred barrier between species had been destroyed, and that some principle of separateness between human and beast had been desecrated.

By contrast, *cross-species transplants are not rejected on any moral grounds by Hindu bioethics.* Hindus believe that God is one with the natural world of multiplicity, and transforms Himself into the ever changing forms of the external world. The Supreme Being is the whole universe, animate and inanimate. This belief supplies the basis for veneration of the natural world that people occupy. Such veneration reaches as far back as the Indus Valley civilization when animals forms were worshipped.

Among animals, special veneration is accorded to the cow, viewed as a goddess, for a specific reason: *the cow is useful to humans* as the source of milk and other necessities. The utility factor does not reduce the animal to an *object*, to be treated as man wills; rather it increases its veneration as a life-giving link in the great chain of life.

The monkey god, Hanumān, celebrated in the Rāmāyaṇa, is worshiped because of his efforts in gaining the release of Sītā, Rāmā's consort, from the captivity of the demon Rāvaṇa. Hanumān is also honored as a fertility God, granting barren women the blessing of children. *The themes throughout are saving and giving life.*

So close is the link between humans and animals in Hinduism that the incarnations of the gods are not limited to human form, as in Christian dogma, but include animal forms. Animals are also portrayed as the vehicles of the gods, as in the case of the lion for Pārvatī; but often the mounts are no more than the gods in animal forms.

In the light of Hinduism's veneration of the natural world, and animals in particular, the religious rejection of animal transplants smacks of Christian *hubris*. Indeed it is considered an affront to man's idea of himself, made in the "image of God," to think that "a piece of animal tissue may occupy the seat of the emotions" and perform efficiently. This is "biological Galileism" and equally humbling. Even so, it is a fact. We are witnessing science confirm the intuition of the ancient Indian sages, that human life is indeed genetically connected with animal life, so to deny that *now* is not just outdated sentimentality, but scientific ignorance. For the most part the old anthropocentricism is harmless, and may be ignored as distinctly quaint, but it becomes positively cruel when conservative Christians sometimes would deny life to a child in order to uphold the biological uniqueness of *homo sapiens*.

At the opposite end of the spectrum from those protesting in behalf of the dignity of the *human recipient*, there were others more concerned with the integrity of the *animal donor*. Animal rights protesters picketed outside Loma Linda University Medical Center against "the use of baboons as organ factories." They failed to impress surgeon Bailey, who said: "I am a member of the human species," meaning: human babies come before baboons.

Hindu bioethics, in the present medical context, would probably agree with the stand of Dr. Bailey, though their rationales are quite different. Hinduism believes that humans occupy the highest life-form, because only humans possess the capacities with which to attain liberation. On this premise, when difficult choices must be made, the Hindu doctor draws on the principle: *human babies come first*. Similar moral reasoning is evident in Caraka, who recommends the consumption of birds and animals for purposes of nutrition; not for the mere titillation of the palate. But since this principle proceeds from a system of thought that is essentially spiritual, and which categorically rejects the Christian *principle of separateness between human and beast*, speceism is given no place. Animals were not made for man, and therefore their integrity must be respected at all times. Only when life is on the line, and priorities must be set, is human life given preference. This is not in the nature of a "donation" but a sacrifice.

SHOULD A BABY BE CONCEIVED TO SAVE A LIFE?

In the summer of 1991, a California teen-ager with a deadly form of leukemia received a transplant of blood-building bone marrow cells from her baby sister, who was conceived in an attempt to save the young woman's life.[5]

Healthy bone marrow, the source of new blood cells, including cells that fight disease, was tapped from the hip of thirteen-month-old Marissa Ayala and given to her sister Anissa, nineteen, at the City of Hope National Medical Center in California.

This was the first time a family had publicly admitted conceiving a child to serve as an organ donor. But many others have done so privately.

Parents have had babies to provide bone marrow for siblings and relatives or even a kidney. Some parents have sought prenatal diagnosis to ensure that the fetus had genetically compatible tissues necessary to serve as a donor, intending to abort if not.

But these parents have shunned publicity, leery of letting the world pry into their ordeals.

In the Ayala's case, their decision to conceive a child as an organ donor was declared in public for all interested parties to examine.

Hindu bioethics examines this case from the point of harm and benefit to all concerned.

From the point of view of the *child*, it is certainly better to have been conceived to donate rather than never to have been conceived at all.

With reference to the *parents*: by conceiving Marissa, the Ayalas were seeking to escape from a desperate dilemma. Their daughter Anissa had chronic myelogenous leukemia, a disease that kills 80 to 90 percent of patients within five years of diagnosis.

Their *daughter's* only hope was a bone marrow transplant. Even then her survival was far from assured—some 20 to 25 percent of patients with marrow transplants die, usually of infections, adverse reactions, or a return of the leukemia.

Upon hearing of Anissa's diagnosis and prognosis, the parents began searching for someone whose tissue type was compatible with hers and who would be willing to donate marrow.

But they could not find a compatible donor. Neither parent had the right tissue type, nor did their son, Airon, who was twenty. A nationwide search for an unrelated donor found none. It was then that the Ayalas decided to conceive a baby as their best hope for finding compatible marrow for Anissa.

Against this background, Hindu bioethics answers the question: *Should a baby be conceived to save her sister?* with the following considerations:

- First, an individuals should be brought into the world and cherished for her own sake and for no other motive.

- Second, the above principle is not amended but added to when the baby that has been conceived can also serve a heroic purpose, *without harm to itself*. In this case, the blessing of life is doubled.
- Third, it follows that the only legitimate purpose for amniocentesis during pregnancy should be to ascertain if the fetal tissues matched, so that the doctor could, on positive finding, save the baby's umbilical cord blood to give along with her marrow when the transplant is administered.
- In the event that the prenatal diagnosis yielded negative results, a decision to terminate the pregnancy would be deemed inhumane. That would clearly demonstrate that the baby had been conceived as a *means to an end*. There is no dilemma here: *it is premeditated murder.*
- On the other hand, even if it were found that the fetus did not have genetically compatible tissues necessary to serve as a donor, Hindu bioethics insists that the child must still be loved and cherished for its own sake.

CHAPTER 6

WHEN PARENTS LET CHILDREN SUFFER FOR REASONS OF FAITH

The American legal system is constantly being placed at odds with the Constitution's guarantee of religious freedom. Quite frequently stories capture headlines, with scenarios such as this. Twelve-year-old "Jody" sits slumped in a chair, her face ashen with pain. She asks a state judge to grant a seemingly suicidal wish: not to have medical treatment for her rare form of bone cancer. Doctors had testified that without chemotherapy and radiation treatment she would die within months. But Jody's father is a minister in a fundamentalist denomination, "The Church Of The Great Physician" (fictitious), that does not permit its members to seek medical treatment and counsels them to rely instead on the power of prayer. Despite her dramatic plea six months ago, the judge ordered hospital care to begin. Her doctor now announces that there is no longer any evidence of the disease. But Jody's father stands firm by his belief in the inefficacy of science and the power of faith. "The medicine didn't do it," he insists. "Jesus healed her. Praise the Lord!"

It is now routine to hear of state courts intervening against the anti-medicine doctrines of some religious groups by ordering treatment for the children of church members when death is imminent. Church history makes it abundantly clear that from its earliest beginnings there have been pious Christians who have regarded recourse to medicine, even in the face of death, as a betrayal of faith. Today, the following four groups stand out officially as defenders of the ancient faith, though many other Christians do so unofficially.

- The Worldwide Church of God, led by Herbert W. Armstrong. He calls vaccines "monkey pus" and likens the use of physicians to worship of pagan gods.

- Christian Science, founded by Mary Baker Eddy (1821–1910). The core of her teachings is the belief that there inheres "no Life, Substance, or Intelligence in matter. That all is mind and there is no matter."[1] With this affirmation Eddy believed she had learned the secret to heal the sick and raise the dead.
- Jehovah's Witnesses, founded by Abel, according to their church history, but led in modern times by Charles Taze Russell (1852–1916). Two publications, *Blood, Medicine and the Law of God* (1961) and *Jehovah's Witnesses and the Question of Blood* 1977), provide the rationales for the Witnesses' refusal to sanction blood transfusion for members of the faith.
- Faith Assembly, headquartered in Indiana. Members are strictly enjoined from using doctors. In a particularly shocking incident in 1981, one-year-old Evie Swanson of Attica, Ind., received second- and third-degree burns when scalding tea spilled over her. Infection set in, was left untreated, and Evie died two days later.

The present situation witnesses a popular revulsion against parents who let their children suffer for reasons of their own faith, and this reaction is moving states to bring charges of neglect or abuse against parents who endanger their children's lives by adhering to religious teachings.

Hindu bioethics approaches these matters of faith and death, guided by three major principles:

1. The Principle of Beneficence
2. The Principle of Parental Authority
3. The Principle of Family Wellbeing

THE PRINCIPLE OF BENEFICENCE

The value of beneficence is deeply embedded in the Hindu culture. Back in Vedic times, we hear the poet ask his companions to 'decorate the Yajña (rite) as they decorate a child to make it look beautiful.' Children are treated with tenderness because they symbolize racial immortality. In the Ṛg Veda a sage prays to Agni: "May I attain immortality with my offspring."[2] Beneficence is later exemplified by the system of *saṁskāras,* or purificatory rites and sacraments.

Among the prenatal *saṁskāras, garbhādhāna* (conception) signifies that concern for the well-being of the child begins with a calculated approach to produce the finest progeny, accompanied by ceremonies that consecrate the child to be. There was the notion that the conduct of the mother influenced the unborn child, therefore the *sīmantonnayana* (hair-parting) rite laid down rules to preserve the physical and mental health of the mother. The best medical knowledge of the day was followed, as Suśruta himself prescribes: "From the time of pregnancy she should avoid coition, over-exertion, sleeping in the day, keeping awake in the night."[3]

Among the *saṁskāras* of childhood, the *Jātakarma* (birth ceremonies) have their origin in the wish to protect the mother and the child and to consecrate the newborn. One item of *Jātakarma* is *Medhājanana*, concerned with the inlellectual well-being of the child; another is *Āyuṣya*, ensuring it a long life.

The *Upanāyana* ceremonies stand out in the educational *saṁskāras*. They provide the youth with a passport into the life of the community, with full rights and responsibilities. They transform his personality so thoroughly that he is ranked as a *dvija* or twice-born.

Even a cursory look at the intent of some of the *saṁskāras* is that the well-being of the child is central, and that this well-being is holistic, incurring no bifurcation between spirit and matter, which could then be made the basis for opposing physical healing to spiritual healing. "It was the business of the Saṁskāras to make the body a valuable possession, a thing not to be discarded, but made holy, a thing to be sanctified, so that it might be a fitting instrument of the spiritual intelligence embodied in it."[4] Thus, the *saṁskāras* serve as a rich repository for constituting the principle of beneficence.

Within the context of the rights of the child to medical care, the principle of beneficence first requires that we prevent harm befalling a child and do our best to promote its physical and emotional well-being. Getting down to details, Terence F. Ackerman says:

> This duty specifically requires that we protect and provide the conditions necessary for a child's physical and mental development. Those conditions include adequate food, clothing, housing, moral training, scholastic education, and opportunities for play and enjoyment. We must protect both physical and mental health and provide freedom from pain and suffering that impairs development. The latter duties of beneficence assume special significance when a child is sick. On the one hand, they suggest the importance of

> providing medical care that may ameliorate the condition. On the other hand, they indicate the importance of witholding interventions that may unnecessarily exacerbate the pain and suffering intrinsic to the disease and its treatment.[5]

The duties of beneficence lie upon the shoulders of parents, physicians, and the state. Parents provide a nurturing environment and are the primary guardians of the child's well-being. Physicians must care for their pediatric patients by preventing any harm befalling them, and by using sound medical judgment to ensure their welfare. Where there are infractions of the law, indicating abuse or neglect on the part of primary caregivers, physicians report such violations to the authorities. The state asserts its interest in the welfare of the child when those who are entrusted with duties of beneficence fail to deliver.

THE PRINCIPLE OF PARENTAL AUTHORITY

A second principle governing the medical care of children is parental authority. In Hinduism, the sinews of parental authority are derived from the makeup of the family. In Dandekar's description: "A Hindu family is normally a closely knit group based on the community of blood, held together by the remarkable affections, the bonds of mutual respect, devotion, and love which develop among various members of a family. This characteristic of the Hindu family is rightly regarded as one of the most beautiful features of the social life of the Hindus."[6]

The authority of the householder ensues from his role as trustee of the legacy bequeathed to him by forefathers and which it is his duty to perpetuate for posterity. The symbol of this historical and cultural continuity is the sacred fire. As keeper of the flame, the householder must perform five great sacrifices: vedic studies; offerings of water to the ancestors; devotional offerings to the gods; offering food to all beings; and extending hospitality. Thus the stature of the householder stems from his being there for all beings dependent upon him, and it is his duty to relate to them in the spirit of sacrifice and service. He gains respect by giving respect.

Given the patriarchal structure of the Hindu home, one is not surprised by the diminished authority of the woman in religious and social terms. Denials of her freedom are piously explained as efforts to protect her. Through the sacrament of marriage she is bonded to her husband and thereafter has no life apart from him. Yet her role is uplifted as mother of the home over which she presides. The bride is told in the wedding hymn (RV, x, 85.46): "Be mistress over thy father-in-law, be mistress over thy mother-in-law." Those words require qualifications, but the fact remains that the solidarity, stability, and moral sensitivity of the family revolve around the housewife. In relationship to her chidren, she is more of a divine entity than father or guru. Śaṁkara points to the source of her authority when he says: "A bad son may be born, but there never is a bad mother."

The child's response to parental authority is unequivocal. The famous "Convocation Address" in the Taittirīya Upaniṣad encapsulates the duty of the child to mother and father. It says:

> Be one to whom a mother is a god.
> Be one to whom a father is a god.[7]

The affirmation of parental authority and filial respect in Hinduism underscores the rights of parents to raise their children in ways they consider best for their physical and personal development. No Hindu would appreciate a Muslim or Christian to dictate appropriate methods of child rearing or suffer social interference in the details of his or her child's care.

Problems arise when parental authority is extended to freedom to allow religious beliefs to determine any or all medical interventions for a child. For example, Jehovah's Witness parents refuse blood transfusion for their children on the grounds that their biblical beliefs (Acts 15:28–29) forbid it and that they are exercising legitimate parental authority by not allowing their children to be transfused, even in life and death situations.

THE PRINCIPLE OF FAMILY WELL-BEING

A third relevant value of Hindu bioethics is embodied in the principle of family well-being. It safeguards beneficence for the family unit, taken as a whole, comprising grandparents, parents, siblings, as well as the sick child. Harmony in the family is prized in Vedic times, and charms were devised to secure it. "Unity of heart, and unity of mind, freedom from hatred do I procure you. Do ye take delight in one another, as a cow in her (new-)born calf!" (AV. VI.III,30.1).

Experts underscore the importance of keeping the family together in the midst of crises. "It is axiomatic in pediatric practice that the physician has a moral duty to support the parents and the family. The diagnosis of a potentially fatal illness in their child places enormous stress upon parents. If parents must contend, in addition, with what they believe to be a transgression of God's law, their ability to function might be further impaired."[8] In addition, perceived stress among parents and family members could produce added stress in the sick child at a time when peace and harmony are essential for the healing process.

A conflict between the principles of beneficence and authority arises when parents, motivated by religious scruples, refuse treatment to their children that might save their lives.

Hindu bioethics attempts to harmonize contending claims in a threefold manner.

First there is full recognition of the rights of parents to make decisions about the health and welfare of their minor children. The state has no business meddling in the way parents take care of their children. Second, this is a *prima facie* right that can be superseded in situations where the parent's exercise of authority poses substantial harm or death to the child. In such life-threatening situations the *prima facie* right can be justifiably removed by action of the state. Third, the principle of beneficence further mandates that the sick child be protected from the burden of pain and suffering. Medical interventions designed to alleviate the child from the consequences of parents' actions should not themselves produce ill effects that exceed the pain and suffering of those actions. In cases where it is probable that the outcome of the intervention that overrides the wishes of the parents for nonintervention will result in a greater degree of substantial harm, then beneficence requires that the course of treatment be witheld. Courts have upheld the rights of chidren who are no longer able to endure the pain and suffering of their treatment to say enough is enough.

For Hindu bioethics, the bottom line in matters of faith and death is that whereas parents have the right freely to practice their faith even to death, that freedom does not extend to putting their children in harm's way. The *vidyārambha* and *upanāyana saṁskāras* demonstrate the value placed on the development of the mind, but until the child reaches the stage of legal discretion, it must not be coerced to becoming a martyr for the faith of its fathers.

The three principles of Hindu bioethics outlined above could be understood as rights, even though in the Hindu cultural context the greater emphasis is on obligations. Interestingly, these principles are affirmed by the

United Nations Convention on the Rights of the Child, with particular reference to Articles 5 and 6. It reads:

Article 5

States Parties shall respect the responsibilities, rights and duties of parents or, where applicable, the members of the extended family. . . to provide, in a manner consistent with the evolving capacities of the child, appropriate direction and guidance in the exercise by the child of the rights recognized in the present Convention.

Article 6

1. States Parties recognize that every child has the inherent right to life.
2. States Parties shall ensure to the maximum extent possible the survival and development of the child.[9]

CHAPTER 7

THE ETHICS OF CONTRACEPTION

The Alan Guttmacher Institute sponsored a study that appeared in the January/February 1988 edition of *Family Planning Perspective,* conveying some good news. It announced that the U.S. rate of unintended pregnancy among women fifteen to forty-four years old is decreasing. And that decline has been accompanied by a decline in the rate of abortions.[1]

Less encouraging was the news that almost half the pregnancies in this country are unintended, and that 54 percent of those "accidents" end in abortion.

Whether they end up in abortion or unplanned birth, unintended pregnancies come at a cost both to the people involved and to society.

Specifically, the rate of unintended pregnancies dropped 16 percent between 1987 and 1994, while the abortion rate declined 11 percent. The unplanned pregnancy rate is highest among eighteen- to twenty-four-year olds and women who are unmarried, low income, black, or Hispanic, the study found.

Moreover, 48 percent of women have had at least one unplanned pregnancy. And 30 percent have had one or more abortions. In 1994 there were 1.4 million abortions in the United States.

Researchers credited the decline in unplanned pregnancies to more effective and wider use of contraceptive methods. They point to a big jump in the use of condoms, particularly in people under age thirty. The key to reducing unplanned pregnancies is decreasing risky behavior and promoting effective contraceptive use.

Opposition to the employment of contraceptives control comes from the Roman Catholic Church. The Vatican permits a married couple to resort to the rhythm method whereby intercourse is limited to the days when the woman biologically cannot conceive a child. The rhythm method is patently one form of birth control. The contention therefore is not with birth control in this broad understanding but with contraception, defined as the use of some means (IUDs, condoms, diaphrams, pills, spermicide, sponge, etc.) to prevent uterine conception.

Official Catholic teaching is found in the encyclical of Pope Pius XI (d. 1939), *Casti Connubi* (1930), which declared:

> Since the conjugal act is destined primarily by nature for the begetting of children, those who in exercising it deliberately frustrate its natural power and purpose sin against nature and commit a deed which is shameful and intrinsically vicious. . . . any use whatsoever of matrimony exercised in such a way that the act is deliberately frustrated in its natural power to generate life is an offense against the law of God and of nature and those who indulge in such are branded with the guilt of grave sin.[2]

Whereas *Casti Connubi* argued that contraception by artificial means is always wrong, other voices in the Catholic Church contended that contraception may be legitimate in certain situations. Pope Paul VI sided with the Church's traditional teachings in his encyclical *Humanae Vitae* ("Of Human Life"), 1968. The key to this document is found in the eleventh paragraph: "the Church calling men back to the observance of the norms of natural law, as interpreted by constant doctrine, teaches that each and every marriage act must remain open to the transmission of life."[3]

The position of Hindu bioethics is closer to the liberal Catholic faction that speaks in terms of "responsible parenthood" than with *Humanae Vitae.*

Hindu bioethics agrees that there are two meanings of the conjugal act: the *unitive* meaning that brings husband and wife together, and the *procreative* meaning that capacitates them for the generation of new lives. It disagrees at the point where the connection between the two meanings is considered "inseparable." Hindu bioethics would argue that the procreative value of the conjugal act need not be bound up with *every* individual act of intercourse. Besides the basic criterion for the meaning of human actions is the total person and not some isolated aspect of the person. Outside Āyurveda's holistic understanding of the agent, the conjugal act appears physiologically structured. If the Church has progressively admitted that a sterile woman may marry and enjoy full conjugal relations, and that intercourse is approved during the so-called safe period, then, Hindu bioethics contends, the next step is to acknowledge that each and every sexual act need not be valued for its fecundity. Humans are not animals. For people, sexual activity is not merely for procreation and gratification, but for expression. We enrich our lives through our sexuality. And contraceptives help free the couple of the anxiety of conceiving an unwanted child. Thus technology enhances the sexual experience. Contraceptive technology is not technology in the sense that an electric toothbrush is technology. The toothbrush cleans my teeth, and that is that. By contrast, contraception simultaneously affects the transmission of life and the act of intercourse that unites two persons in passion and in love. By eliminating anxiety in the possibility of conception, it adds to the pleasure of the experience.

Indians have sought such sexual freedom from earliest times. The Brihadāraṇyaka Upaniṣad states:

> Now, the woman whom one may desire with the thought, "May she not conceive offspring!"—after inserting the member in her and joining mouth with mouth, he should first inhale, and then exhale, and say: "With power, with semen, I reclaim the semen from you!" Thus she comes to be without seed.[4]

The effectiveness of the above method may leave one questioning; however, there is no doubt about the use of contraceptives in early Indian society. Ethicist Seshagiri Rao states:

> Generally, Hindus show little resistance to the idea of birth control. There is no objection to contraception on religious or moral grounds. . . . A temperate exercise of sex instinct by the householder is recommended in the *sāśtras* (religious treatises) themselves; and contraception helps in avoiding unwanted and undesirable pregnancies. Hence contraception is generally acceptable to the Hindus and is to be encouraged in the interests of domestic felicity and welfare of society.[5]

The problem facing the Hindu bioethicist is more complex than establishing acceptance for use of contraceptives; it involves the need for a variety of contraceptive methods. Harking back to the Guttmacher report cited earlier, consider: 58 percent of women who had an abortion reported they had used a contraceptive the month they became pregnant, as did 48 percent who had unplanned births.

That underscores the need for a variety of contraceptive methods, such as: hormonal, shots, oral, barriers, implants, IUDs, and access to male and female sterilization. The Hindu bioethicist would wish to learn all facts connected to each method. She would definitely reject those birth-control devices that might cause harm to the woman, including resort to abortion.

By way of *practical* example, Hindu bioethics would be comfortable endorsing a birth-control device, such as the FDA-approved implant, sold under the brand name of Norplant. It is cheaper than the pill and nearly as reliable as sterilization (annual failure rate is well below 1 percent). It is just a way of delivering progestin, an antifertility hormone contained in birth-control pills. Six small capsules are implanted under the armpit. They slowly release progestin. The hormone blocks ovulation and keeps sperm out of the uterus by thickening the cervical mucus.

Hindu bioethics endorses such technologies, because they not only function as safe, reliable methods of contraception, but nurture family bonds through ties of intimacy.

Hindu bioethics also emphasizes the need to educate people to use contraceptives correctly and consistently. Providers must spend time with patients, counseling, answering questions, and explaining risks, side effects, and proper usage.

For women from low-income families, the state would find it cheaper to provide them with free contraceptives than to incur hefty expenses for welfare cases later on. Āyurveda would enthusiastically support all such efforts as part of its preventive approach in matters of public health.

CHAPTER 8

THE ETHICS OF PRENATAL DIAGNOSIS FOR SEX SELECTION

THE BOY-GIRL TEST

In a typical Indian household, a mother of two daughters is very happy when she knows she is going to have a son. It could mean an end to taunts of her mother-in-law and neighbors. She will gain "honor" by having a boy.

The pregnant woman is certain this time around it is a boy, because she has had an amniocentesis test, popularly known as "the boy-girl test." Though it is clinically intended to detect congenital deformities, the test is socially employed as a means for sex selection.

The procedure involves the withdrawal by a long hypodermic needle of a small sample of the amniotic fluid that bathes the fetus in the womb. The fluid contains cells that have flaked off the fetus. The chromosomes in these cells can be examined for evidence of birth defects, but they also tell the sex of the fetus. The test is totally accurate, but costs thousands of rupees.

A second sex discrimination test is ultrasound. The machine takes a picture of the fetus in the sixteenth week of pregnancy, which tells the sex of the child. It is not completely accurate, but costs much less.

In the event that the test proves "negative"—meaning another girl—there is a strong likelihood that a family with two daughters will opt for an abortion.

Seema Sirohi reports: "There are no definite numbers on how many abortions occur after such tests. One authoritative study said 78,000 female fetuses were aborted from 1978 to 1983 nationwide following sex-discrimination tests."[1]

Doctors who run the lucrative businesses say it is better to abort a female fetus than to subject an unwanted child to a life of suffering. In the opinion of one doctor who runs New Delhi's most popular boy-girl testing clinic: "People are willing to keep producing children until they get a son. Tell me, is it not better to let them have a chance so they don't have six daughters before they have a son? Either you should educate the masses that there is no difference between sons and daughters or give them a choice. This test, in fact, is helping the population-control program of the government."[2]

For the masses, there is indeed a "difference between sons and daughters." In India sons are looked upon as potential wage earners, as support for parents in old age, and as performers of rituals for ancestors. On the other hand, multiple daughters can pose as financial liabilities, especially when it comes to marriage expenses. A developing consumer society has increased demands for dowry, from the traditional jewelry to cars, refrigerators, even houses. According to Sundari Nanda, head of the New Delhi police department's Crime Against Women Cell: "We are becoming a very materialistic and consumer-driven society. For such a society, dowry becomes a way of betterment for those in the process of climbing up."[3]

In India's rush to embrace modernity, the demand for dowry has become a lever for extorting money and goods from a bride's family for years after the wedding. If her family does not comply, she frequently is subjected to cruelty, physical abuse, and often death.

Police say reported dowry deaths have increased 170 percent nationwide in the last decade, with 6,200 recorded in 1994—an average of 17 married women burned, poisoned, strangled, or otherwise killed each day because of their family's failure to meet the dowry demands of the husband's family.[4] More recently, *The Hindustan Times* reports "Dowry-related violence claims 5,000 victims every year."[5]

It is commonly believed that the statistics represent only a fraction of the actual cases believed to have been committed. They also do not include the tens of thousands of incidents of nonfatal dowry harassment and physical and mental abuse inflicted on wives by husbands and in-laws.

Hindu bioethcs finds the prenatal sex discrimination tests a perverted use of modern science. It is a scarcely concealed form of female feticide. It is the employment of modern technology to perpetuate ancient social prejudices against women.

The moral arguments often heard that it is not fair to bring little girls into the world who are going to suffer, because their families do not want them, or that the tests help the population-control programs of the government, are all specious. If *dayā* is informed by such convoluted logic, it follows that it is better to kill all rejects of society, rather than to allow these unwanted victims to suffer rejection, poverty, and deprivation. This gives a barbaric twist to the concept of *preventive medicine.* The cure is worse than the disease.

Hindu bioethics supports legislation to ban amniocentesis as a prenatal sex discrimination test, when utilized as a means of female feticide. In principle it supports the enactment of laws that would provide for:

1. Prohibition of the misuse of prenatal diagnostic techniques for determination of the sex of the fetus, leading to female feticide
2. Prohibition of advertising of prenatal diagnostic techniques to determine sex
3. Permission and regulation of the use of prenatal diagnostic techniques to detect specific genetic abnormalities or disorders
4. Permission for the use of such techniques only under certain conditions by registered institutions
5. Punishment for violations of these provisions

However, it would be terribly naive to think that legislation can end sex-discrimination tests. Two truths about the marketplace are: if a demand exists, it will be supplied; and you cannot ban a proven technology out of existence. Also, ones who feel the cost of banning most are the poor; the rich resort to private clinics.

What is really needed is education and the social awareness that comes with it. The reason why we do not hear of dowry deaths in Kerala is because it is India's most literate state. *The New Education Policy,* which was approved by Parliament in 1986, has devoted a full chapter on women's education and how to implement it. The report says that between 1951 and 1981, the percentage of literacy among women improved from 7.93 percent to 24.82 percent. However, in absolute numbers, illiterate women have increased during this period from 158.7 million to 241.7 million. According to the 1981 census, 248 women out of every 1,000 are educated, compared to 469 men.

In addition to literacy, social standing, and economics, Hindu bioethics sees the need for the improvement of women's health. Life expectancy for Indian women has gone up from 20.3 years in 1901 to 40.6 years in 1951 to 50 years in 1971 and 54.7 years in 1981. Since 1971, the gap between the life expectancy of women has almost been bridged.[6] Āyurveda is particularly sensitive to the connection between health and environment. Hindu bioethics therefore calls for more research on the impact of environmental degradation on women's reproductive health.

Finally, Hindu bioethics finds need for a new image of women. Already India's 330 million women have traveled far from their traditional image, which received religious and social acceptability to keep women illiterate, to confine them to the four walls of the home, and to treat them as the property of men. Regrettably, the medical manuals have shades of this traditional image, which is to acknowledge that its science is always in tension with culture. However, practice aside, the principles of Hindu bioethics have all of the humanistic elements to make for a new image of the Indian woman—

- A woman who does not accept that biology is destiny and that karma is king
- A woman who sees herself as different but equal to men
- A woman who honors herself as an individual, having her own dignity
- A woman who accepts her body as good, beautiful, and a source of happiness
- A woman who reacts to her miserable situation in society; who gets angry, and fights back against the odds

Thus Hindu bioethics focuses on *the person and the image of the person* as cause and cure of the problem of dowry deaths. It is indeed ironical that a tradition, originally intended for daughters in a culture where women were not entitled to family inheritances, should have evolved into an insidious practice that legitimates theft through marriage, that bankrupts families, and that threatens the lives of women from the moment their sex is known within the privacy and sanctity of the womb. At this point *clinical use* succumbs to *social abuse*—a gross parody of means and ends.

CHAPTER 9

THE ETHICS OF THE HUMAN GENOME PROJECT

The doctor's office is already beginning to wear a new look. Alongside the traditional diplomas and pictorial renderings of skeletal parts and organs, we see colorful charts that depict the twenty-three pairs of human chromosomes and pinpoint on each one the location of the genes that can predispose people to serious disease. The charts signify the completion of the Human Genome Project. Begun in 1988, this multibillion dollar government-sponsored effort has two basic aims:

1. To identify the 100,000 genes packed into the human genome, the strand of DNA in the nucleus of each of the body's 100 trillion cells;

and

2. To sequence, or place in order, the 3 billion chemical code letters in that strand, thus giving scientists "the ability to read natures's complete blueprint for creating a human being."[1]

Francis Collins, Director of the Human Genome Project, is not speaking hyperbolically when he estimates it as "dwarfs going to the moon." Determining the order and organization of all this genetic material has been compared to "tearing six volumes of the *Encyclopaedia Brittanica* into pieces, then trying to put it all back together to read the information." Yet scientists consider it worth the effort, because the knowledge gained from it will radically impact all areas of our lives: sciences, industry, law, agriculture, environment. Most of all it will revolutionize the practice of medicine.

Down the road, doctors will be able to give us DNA fingerprints of genes that predispose us to common kinds of diseases by extracting DNA from the blood of newborn infants and then mechanically analyzing 100 or so genes. A computer will be able to read the genetic profile and dispense medical directives. Geneticist Mark Skolnick of the University of Utah explains: "Once you can make a profile of a person's genetic predisposition to disease, medicine will finally become largely predictive and preventive."[2]

Other ways in which the genetic blueprint for humans will revolutionize the practice of medicine will include: new classes of drugs; new kinds of treatments; new definitions of disease, based on underlying genetic defects, not on overt symptoms. "Armed with a patient's genetic data, doctors may someday be able to diagnose diseases before they occur or prescribe medications custom-made to fit each patient's unique genetic profile."[3]

ETHICAL IMPLICATIONS OF THE HUMAN GENOME PROJECT

Hindu bioethics supports the Human Genome Project for its efforts toward expanding our understanding of human biology and disease, especially because this knowledge will be *universally applicable* to benefit human health. Genetic knowledge will not only free future generations of killer diseases, but will give us the tools to reshape the human experience. Hindu bioethics lauds the program for publishing its results on the Web, free to all comers.

Nearer to its philosophy of medicine, Hindu bioethics welcomes the project's role toward setting the stage for:

- A new era of *preventive medicine*
- New insights to treat each *patient as a person*, having a unique genetic profile
- New confirmation for Āyurveda's *karmic stance* that we need not remain hapless victims of our destiny but can do something toward overcoming our inherited past

Hindu bioethics does not view these developments as a case of *man playing God*, but as of *God playing man*. A cardinal belief of Hinduism is that the Supreme Being manifests itself in evolutionary form. Matter struggles with Spirit, but Spirit, stage by stage, comes into its own. The

Bhadvadgītā says: "Unmanifest is the origin of beings, manifest their mid-most stage, and unmanifest again their end."[4] We are here—in the "*mid-most stage.*" This understanding of cosmic process as the arena in which *Spirit is progressively and innovatively expressed* makes the Hindu philosophic vision open and adaptable to all of the wondrous promises of genetic science, even as it wields a god-like capacity to deliver the very blueprint for human life.

However, we are not yet in the promised land. The Human Genome Project has sparked global interest in a large array of questions pertaining to the ethical, legal, and social implications of the existence and use of human genetic sequences. Though the forms of the questions raised in respect to the accessibility and increase of information are novel to the emerging technology, they express familiar ethical concerns. "The volume, variety, and the ease with which such information can be obtained, and the vast number of people affected, make it imperative that the possible use or misuse of the project's findings be anticipated and addressed."[5]

Hindu bioethics addresses two major concerns.

First, we all know that in a competitive marketplace, employers want full productivity from their workers, and might therefore choose to select employees with the assistance of genetic screening. Two questions that arise are: do employers have the right to reject candidates on the basis of genetic findings, and do prospective employees have the right to refuse to be screened?

Similar thinking could govern the insurance policies of Health Management Organizations (HMOs). Clients with histories of hereditary diseases would be considered high risks and would therefore be charged exorbitant premiums, while other such individuals may be totally rejected as uninsurable. HMOs might argue that they have a right to genetic data for their actuarial tables in order to function as viable businesses.

In both instances, Hindu bioethics would reject claims of the workplace and insurance companies for genetic disclosures on the grounds of its principles of privacy, confidentiality, ownership, and autonomy. These principles must determine who should have access to the *genetic information* and under what circumstances; and what rights, if any, employers, insurers, and family members have to an individual's genetic profile. Moreover, Hindu bioethics would support legislation to protect people at risk against *genetic discrimination* in health insurance and employment.

Second, there is the dilemma of giving or witholding full genetic information by a doctor to a patient. Here much depends on how powerful the information is. Huntington's disease provides a good example. It is invariably fatal after a horrible decline. If a doctor tells somebody he or she has that variation of the gene, the physician has given the already traumatized individual more information than can be rationally and emotionally assimilated. The situation becomes particularly problematic in situations where the diagnoses of genetic disorders are available *prior to the availability of treatments*. Caraka's guidelines suggest discretionary disclosure, keeping in mind the capacity of the individual patient and family to "take it" and to profit by it. Of course, an underlying assumption of this line of Indian thought is that the doctor knows the patient and family intimately; a quality of relationship that is not always obtainable in America's big cities.

It is worth noting that until genetic information became available, it was an axiom of the new medicine in the United States to require full disclosure, and to categorically dub the conditional approach of Caraka and company as paternalistic and outdated; but now the availability of genetic information has dramatically changed all that. It is quite revealing that while a diagnostic test for Huntington's disease has been available for some time, most people at risk decline to take it. It seems that, for many, the cost of knowing too much about their genetic endowment is a psychological price too high to pay.

In the modern West, the most serious implications of genetic testing have less to do with employers and insurers and more to do with members of one's own family. Questions arise: "Will marital bonds be stressed when newlyweds discover that a spouse has the Huntington's disease variation? How will a parent feel who has given his offspring the disease? How do you tell your children you may have given a killer-disease to them?" In a culture in which death is still a taboo subject, both in the medical profession and in the population at-large, such queries take ominous form.

These questions are most painful when we focus on rare diseases like Huntington's, where the errant gene seals an inescapable fate. But the infrequency of such diseases does not make for a proper model for understanding the impact of *most genetic information*. The bottom line is that in the majority of cases, genes only predict *susceptibility* to diseases, not *certainty*. This element of conditionality gives clinical support to Caraka's model of karma, which urges medical intervention and resists succumbing to fatalistic predictions.

CHAPTER 10

THE ETHICS OF GENETIC ENGINEERING

A new revolution is sweeping medicine. The *first* revolution in Western medicine occurred in 1854, when British surgeon John Snow discovered that cholera was spread by contaminated water, ushering systems of sanitation that saved millions from deadly infections. The *second* revolution also happened toward the end of the nineteenth century, with the use of anesthesia in surgery, which made it possible for surgeons to perform operations within the body cavity, as in the case of appendicitis. The *third* revolution saw the arrival of vaccines and antibiotics, which helped prevent or cure a host of infectious diseases. For all these strides, Western medicine has at best remedied infectious diseases and some surgical problems, but it has not "cured" anything. Drugs and surgery make it possible for the body to heal itself; they relieve symptoms without rectifying the underlying problems. The *fourth* medical revolution promises to change all of that. It is the genetic revolution, armed with new technologies that will enable us to improve on nature. Dr. W. French Anderson, a pioneer of human genetic engineering and indeed "the father of gene therapy," predicts that within thirty years, there will be a gene-based therapy for most diseases. Human genetic engineering will not only profoundly change the practice of medicine, but will impact every aspect of our culture. The big question it poses for ethics is: *How far should we go?*

Human genetic engineering or gene therapy is based on an understanding of the body in which genes provide the system of defense and healing. Genes protect the body, repair damage, and restore it to health. As with the *doṣa* theory of disease in Āyurveda, when genes become abnormal they not only produce "genetic" diseases, such as sickle-cell anemia and Huntington's disease, but can also contribute to cancer and heart disease.

Hence, Anderson's final solution: "If we want to cure a disease, therefore, we must do it at the level of the genes."[1]

The movement to fight diseases with altered or new genes is just beginning. In 1990 the Human Gene Therapy Subcommittee (HGTS) approved the first gene therapy protocol. It was from Michael Blaese and French Anderson for gene therapy on children, including Ashanti De Silva, who suffer from severe combined immunodeficiency (SCID), often called the "bubble-boy" disease, because its most famous victim was encased in a plastic bubble during his short life to protect him from infection. One form of SCID called ADA deficiency is caused by a defect that blocks production of adenosine deaminase, a key enzyme; without it, important immune-system blood cells are immobilized.

In a speech delivered here in Honolulu,[2] at which the author was present, Blaese described how his team at the NIH, in September 1990, performed successful gene therapy on Ashanti "Ashi" De Silva, now a normal teenager. Four months later, the group performed the same therapy on Cindy Cutshall, then nine.

Both girls were afflicted with ADA. Because of a flawed gene, the T-cells of their immune system were not able to produce ADA, the enzyme necessary for their survival.

To treat the children, the NIH team took viruses from mice, engineered them to remove the genes, then replaced them with normal ADA genes.

Though the experiment was novel and brilliant, Blaese and fellow scientists knew that the girls had been *treated* but *not cured.* Altered blood cells survive only for a few months, necessitating repetitions of the procedure. To effect a complete cure, gene therapists would have to get to the source of the problem: the long-lasting stem cells that reside in bone marrow and produce all the white blood cells that circulate in the bloodstream.

And that is precisely what Blaese did. He inserted healthy ADA genes into stem cells drawn out of Ashi's bone marrow. He then inserted the altered cells into the bloodstream, hoping they would find their way back to the marrow.

In an informal interview with a Honolulu reporter, Blaese said:

> We're still very early in development of this treatment, but worldwide, several thousand patients have received gene therapy directed at one or another disorder.
>
> A whole series of gene therapies for cancer are going through clinical trials and other trials are under way.

> Genes are the sets of instructions that direct the function and structure of all living things, so when you have a disease that is caused by a garbled set of instructions, which is really what genetic diseases are, the most elegant way to treat them would be to put in a new set of instructions. *That is basically gene therapy.*[3]

HOW FAR SHOULD WE GO?

Hindu bioethics distinguishes between (1) somatic cell gene therapy and (2) enhancement genetic engineering.

(1) In terms of *somatic cell gene therapy,* we have seen that many diseases, such as ADA deficiency, and also sickle-cell anemia, hemophilia, and Gaucher disease, are caused by a defect in a single gene. In all such cases, Hindu bioethics supports treatment on the grounds of its *principle of beneficence.* The patients are desperately ill, or they are facing the attack of a monstrous illness, so everything must be done to relieve suffering. Gene therapy is their only hope. To be sure, there are risks involved. Cutting-edge medical research is always risky, but, relative to the severe privations and certain death, the risks and uncertainties of gene therapy are at acceptable levels. A report says:

> For the most part, the specter of Frankenstein creations escaping from the laboratory has been quelled by carefully monitored, slowly progressing research. Civic, religious, scientific, and medical groups have all agreed in principle that somatic-cell gene therapy is appropriate for humans (11, U.S. Congress. Office of Technology Assessment 1984, p. 47).[4]

The Hindu values that are salient in support of this therapy is the familial *principle of obligation* to ensure survival of present and future generations. Hindu bioethics has no special problem with death, but with *premature death,* and we know so many children like Ashanti DeSilva and Cindy Cutshall desperately need treatment.

Mistakes are bound to be made, because we are dealing here with the development of complex technology. The death of Jesse Gelsinger, an eighteen year old, suffering with a rare liver disorder is a case in point. His death in September 1999 was the first ever linked to gene therapy. It served to humble medicine's best and brightest at the University of Pennsylvania. Scientists met before a NIH panel to determine what went wrong with this young man and how to make certain it does not happen again. A mother and her son traveled to this meeting to relay to the scientists the simple words of her seventeen-year-old boy, Brett, who has the same liver disorder. He said: "Mom, please tell them I want to have gene therapy. I hate being sick. I want to be normal."[5]

Hindu bioethics supports the use of gene transfer treatment for serious diseases that prevent children from leading normal lives by keeping them in constant pain and sending them to an early death. Victims of cancer, viral diseases such as AIDS, and some forms of cardiovascular diseases are all considered appropriate candidates for treatment.

(2) Somatic cell gene therapy also has the potential for *enhancement genetic engineering*—"for supplying a specific characteristic that individuals might want for themselves (somatic cell engineering) or their children (germline engineering) which would not involve the treatment of a disease."[6] The slide from correction to perfection is already under way. For example, the human-growth hormone was devised for chidren with prospects of growing up the size of dwarfs, but it was soon used by children who only *though*t they were "dwarfs" for their age and were blessed with wealthy parents who could pay $30,000 for a year's treatment of growth hormones.

Hindu bioethics believes there is a medical and moral divide between *somatic cell gene therapy* and *enhancement genetic engineering*, which must not be crossed, and which serves as a marker for how far genetic engineering should go at this stage of development.

Discussion of the pros and cons of this stance was recently precipitated by a report in the journal *Nature* of a new study that sheds light on how memory works and raises questions pertaining to the morality of using genetics to make people brainier.[7]

Scientists at Princeton, M.I.T., and Washington University succeeded in altering the DNA of mice so as to change the reactions between neurons deep within the cranium. These genetically engineered animals appeared ordinary, but in lab tests involving learning and memory they proved they are "whizzes" that could learn more rapidly, remember for longer times, and adapt to environmental changes more resiliently than normal mice. The result is a new strain of mice, smarter than their "dim-witted cousins." The scientists declared that their results suggest that the genetic enhancement of mental and cognitive attributes such as intelligence and memory in mammals is feasible.[8]

In the short run, the scientists established a theory about how brain synapses make connections and store knowledge, but the research also anticipated the day when genetic adjustment of memory and intelligence will be possible for humans.

That day may not be so far-fetched. Today doctors can screen fetuses for genetic diseases; tomorrow they will be able to correct the problem in utero. But a boundary is crossed when doctors move from *treatment to enhancement.*

So far as *therapeutic possibilities* are concerned, Hindu bioethics is on the side of progress. We should hope that this research may lead to practical medical results for humans, targeting learning and memory disorders among older people, including Alzheimer's disease. However, there is a difference between using such treatment to reverse an elderly person's Alzheimer's disease and helping a college student get an 'A' in an exam. It is one thing for a boy to want to be on par with his classmates to compete in high school basketball; it is another thing for a boy to receive human-growth hormones because the latest teenage fad is: "I want to be like Mike"—legendary superstar of the Chicago Bulls. The difference is between *values* and *vanity*. This divide between *correcting* and *perfecting* gives rise to many ethical quandaries, which Hindu bioethics confronts.

First, a fact that must be reckoned with is that *self-improvement* is as much of an American religion as being Baptist. Hindu bioethics has no trouble with that, as long as one has a clear notion of the *nature of the self* that is to be improved. Arguing from one view of the self, a person can legitimately say, "There is absolutely no difference between getting one's child the *best school* (dream of all normal parents and the nightmare of the Japanese), and getting one's child a *perfect gene*. What is the big fuss?"

The answer of bioethicist Erik Parens of the Hastings Center is that there is a difference, and it has to do with the difference "between cultivating and purchasing capacities."[9] Buying a Harvard education could very well enhance a child's natural gifts, but it is different from buying the capacities. The Bhagavadgītā says much the same:

> Let a man lift himself by himself; let him not degrade himself; for the Self alone is the friend of the self [person] and the Self alone is the enemy of the self.[10]

The meaning of the Gītā *for us* is that divinity in all its richness resides within the ordinary self, and that it can work for us (friend) or against us (enemy), depending on how much it is part of our consciousness. *There is no stasis in nature.* Personal transformation is a function of the inner life—seeing with the "third eye" is not an acquisition of reconstructive laser surgery. To uplift oneself, one must therefore engage creative forces that are within and not simply rely on appendages that can be purchased at a price. In brief: *self improvement is improvement of the self.*

Second, on medical grounds, Hindu bioethics proceeds on the principle: "Do no harm." Somatic cell enhancement engineering threatens human values because our limited knowledge makes it risky business. As a pioneer in this field, geneticist Anderson's words of caution are worth heeding. He acknowledges that we have rough ideas of how simple genes work, and that there are thousands of "housekeeping genes" that do the job of running cells, yet our understanding is limited when it comes to how an organ develops into its particular size and shape. Similarly, we know how the nervous system works, in terms of electric circuits, memory storage, and transmission of signals; yet we are far removed from understanding thought and consciousness, to say nothing of the "spiritual side of our existence."[11]

Though we have few clues as to how a thinking, loving, interacting organism can be derived from its molecules, the day is coming when we can change some of those molecules. This prospect leaves Anderson worried. There are probably genes that influence the brain's organization, structure, metabolism, and circuitry, making possible a human's capacity to think abstractly, morally, and existentially. Mathematics, ideas of good and evil, anticipations of death, and visions of 'God' are all involved. But "what if in our innocent attempts to improve our genetic makeup we alter one or more of those genes? Could we test for the alteration? Certainly not at present. If we caused a problem that would affect the individual or his or her offspring, could we repair the damage? Certainly not at present. Every parent who has several children knows that some babies accept and give more affection than others, in the same environment. Do genes control this? What if these genes were accidentally altered? How would we even know if such a gene were altered?"[12]

Third, Hindu bioethics responds to enhancement engineering with reference to its *principle of consequentialism.* It is axiomatic to the Indian mind that everything has its own store of karma that eventually plays itself out. Enhancement research, as just mentioned, is not at that point that we know all outcomes—*Frankenstein* movies always warn the jittery audience, "These experiments may not go as originally planned." It would not be a scare tactic to say that parents would be making decisions on bahalf of their children over which they had no control and whose long-term effects would be uncertain or even dangerous. Who can predict all side effects? Can we be certain that a child engineered to become intellectually sharp could actually turn out morally mean? What happens when the 'supermice' get old? Scientists already fear that altered mice might be more prone to strokes, chronic pain, and premature death. There are other possible complications indicating that it may not be wise to try to fool Mother Nature.

Fourth, Hindu bioethics appeals to the *principle of justice*, based on our common spiritual heritage. All life comes from one universal source called *Parameṣwara*. The Bhagavadgītā says: "When one sees Me everywhere and everything in Me, I am never lost to him and he is never lost to Me" (VI.30). This thought invests each individual with equality, and raises questions of social fairness. Do we wish to usher in a society where the rich get smarter? Who will have a right to access to the technology once it becomes financially out of reach for the common person? Every parent would want his or her child to be intellectually enhanced, but only a minority would be able to afford it. Would this not create a new 'caste system' in which the wealthy brāhmins of society look down upon those children who are not enhanced, because they have lower IQs?

Fifth, even if the fairness question were resolved, is enhancing our abilities medically sound? The Āyurvedic view that health must be understood in terms of the *principle of balance* suggests that changes brought about by genetic engineering in one area could adversely affect balance in other areas. UCLA neurobiologist Alcino Silva argues, "Everything comes at a price. Very often when there's a genetic change where we improve something, something else gets hit by it, so it's never a clean thing."[13] With more alarm, Jeremy Rifkin asks: "How do you know you're not going to create a mental monster? We may be on the road to programming our own extinction."[14]

Sixth, the pluralistic approach of Hindu ethics values diversity and finds richness in individuality devised by the evolutionary wisdom of Mother Nature who does not put all of her eggs in one basket. Therefore the prospects of a homogenized society, shaped by certain dominant traits and values, is a little frightening.

Seventh, Hindu bioethics adopts an inclusive approach toward humans and other forms of beings; unlike the Western approach that limits genetic engineering to human considerations, and human concerns. Harold Coward makes our point:

> Proponents of genetic engineering often look at the process of animal engineering and its results strictly from the human perspective—from the bene-

> fits that will accrue to humans. For example, genetically engineered "super pigs and chickens" may increase the amount of food for human consumption. But what about the effect upon the animals themselves. Or consider medical research. Animals are genetically engineered to model some of the most devastating diseases that afflict humans. To accomplish this goal, however, requires that large numbers of animals live lives of intense pain and suffering. The ethics of inflicting such suffering upon animals so as to potentially benefit humans has received little attention in the West.[15]

Hindu bioethics addresses the genetic engineering of animals from the perspectives of three principles: (1) unity; (2) interconnectedness; and (3) interdependence.

(1) The *principle of unity* is formed on the basis of the notion that Supreme Being cosmically manifests itself in evolutionary terms. All levels of existence are manifestations of a single Reality. It is the same evolving Spirit that ascends from the level of consciousness in the animal kingdom, to the level of intelligence in the kingdom of humans. Therefore, while there is a distinction between humans and animals, there is no separation. Humans are intrinsically related to animals, as parts of nature, and hence there can be no basis for pretensions of dominance. Philosophically, the unitive worldview of Hindu ethics avoids the dichotomy present in Western religious, philosophic, and scientific thinking between men and animals, and the exploitation that justifies.

(2) The philosophic principle of oneness sets the stage for viewing animal and human processes in terms of *the principle of interconnectedness*. Animals and humans belong to one web of life. Being connected, all forms of life impact one another, hence the importance of acknowledging the consequences of human actions on animal life forms.

(3) Third, since life is one, and all of its myriad parts are interconnected, it follows that the model of our relationships with animals must rest on *the principles of interdependence* and *reciprocity*. For example, pharmacists have used the venom of the Brazilian pit viper to develop Capoten for high blood pressure, among hundreds of other such remedies. Caraka lists animals and birds as important medical resources. The place given to the cow in Indian culture is the best-known example of interdependence. Gandhi held to the view that "Cow protection is the gift of Hinduism to the world. It is a distinctive contributiion to the world's religious ideas." Gandhi scholar Seshagiri Rao explains that, for Gandhi, 'cow' meant the entire subhuman world, and stands for the protection of

the weak and helpless.[16] The principle of "cow protection" says to humans: Because you are smarter and stronger, you are doubly obligated to do good by creatures that are less endowed. Thus, for Hindu bioethics: *privilege entails responsibility* or, as the French have it: noblesse oblige. Moral stakes are all the more enhanced when *responsibility* is reinforced by *reciprocity*.

CHAPTER 11

THE ETHICS OF CLONING

In the beginning there was Dolly. *The Observer* broke the news to a stunned world that on July 5, 1996, Scottish scientist Ian Wilmut, of the Roslin Institute, had cloned a sheep named Dolly. Results were published in the British journal *Nature*, March 1997. Wilmut explained that he had replaced the genetic material of a sheep's egg with the DNA from an adult sheep and created a lamb that is a clone of the adult.

While other researchers had previously produced genetically identical animals by dividing embryos soon after they had been formed by eggs and sperm, Wilmut was the first to create a clone using DNA from an adult animal.

Wilmut reported that as a source of genetic material, he had used udder or mammary cells from a six-year-old sheep. The cells were put into tissue culture and manipulated to make their DNA become quiescent.

Then Wilmut removed the nucleus, containing the genes, from an egg cell taken from another ewe. He fused that egg cell with one of the adult udder cells.

When the two cells merged, the genetic material from the adult took up residence in the egg and directed it to grow and divide. Wilmut implanted the developing embryo in a third sheep, who gave birth to a healthy lamb that is a clone of the adult that provided its DNA.

In numerous interviews Wilmut has said he wanted to create new animals that could be used for medical research, and has dismissed the notion of cloning humans.

He acknowledges there is no reason in principle why it cannot be done, but hastens to add, "All of us would find that offensive."[1]

Dolly is now history. In the meteoric world of reproductive biology, University of Hawaii professor Ryuzo Yanagimachi and his thirty-one-year-old postdoctoral student, Teruhiko Wakayama, succeeded in making dozens of copies of a mouse and thus taking cloning "one step closer the assembly line."

Yanagimachi followed Wilmut's technique, and then decided to innovate on two counts: (1) instead of using electric shocks to coax an adult cell into merging with the host egg, whose nucelus had been removed, Yanagimachi injected just the adult nucleus into a nucleus-free host; (2) he then let the hybrid cell sit for up to six hours before stimulating it to start dividing. Result: the University of Hawaii team was able to make more than fifty copies of a mouse, three generations in all. The cloned mice showed all signs of normalcy—could mate; give birth; and their DNA was strong and healthy to the point that they themselves could be cloned, and their own clones cloned!

A year after their success in cloning three generations of female mice in 1997, the University of Hawaii team had another breakthrough, proving that males can be cloned too, and thus ending the all-girls club of cloned animals. Fibro, a male mouse, was cloned, without using cells from a female animal's reproductive system, suggesting that animals can be cloned from any cell in the body. Fibro was created from cells taken from a male mouse's tail. Up to this point, researchers had thought that cloning male animals would be more difficult than females, but the UH research shows that there is no difference.

The research of the University of Hawaii scientists, along with the work of many others all over the world, is "one giant step for mankind," hastening the day for complete human cloning. We witness today how the fiction of one decade becomes the technology of another. Lawmakers will make stump speeches and pass legislation that cuts off federal funds, but human-cloning research will go underground and, with private entrepreneurial support, emerge only when they have succeeded. Bioethicist Daniel Callahan predicts: "I don't see how you can stop these things. We are at the mercy of these technological developments. Once they're here, it's hard to turn back."[2]

Scientists pretend that they do not know the time or place of *homo sapiens'* 'second coming,' but some science observers who read the signs of the times fear it will be soon. A new Adam or Eve could come shrieking into the world within five years. If that prophecy is correct, science had better get its ethical house in order, quickly.

In an article, "Playing God," *Hinduism Today* squarely faced some of the ethical issues connected with human cloning by canvassing the opinions of a variety of Hindu leaders. After alluding to the creation of Raktabīja ("blood drop"), replicated on the battlefield in drops of blood; the creation of Lord Gaṇesha from the skin of his mother and Lord Murugan by a spark from Śiva's third eye, and so on, the article acknowledges "there is no easily found scripture directly addressing the practice of cloning," and therefore we must rely on "induction and extrapolation."[3]

Mata Amritanandamayi, "President of Hinduism" (*sic*) at the Parliament of the World's Religions, 1993, said: "The idea of cloning, though implemented only recently through modern science, was in the minds of the ancient saints and sages of India." This type of response is typical of orthodox Hindus who confuse mythology with history. Caraka would reject such thinking on rational grounds.

Chakrapani Ullal of the American Association of Vedic Astrologers claims that religious sanctification of marriage helps ensure the birth of high souls; lacking that, "people born through cloning will be fraught with problems." Such thinking (which would be offensive to the Pāṇḍavas) makes ritual into magic and is antithetical to Āyurveda's clinical approach to scientific issues.

Mrs. Ullal states that a normal being cannot be born from a "conception" devoid of love. The 2,000-year-old *Tirumantram* appears to support such thinking, "describing how each embodied soul is influenced by the consciousness and energies of the parents before and during coitus." True, but we are talking about "duties in distress," which, like *niyoga*, was permitted if practiced as a passionless act. Moreover, Hinduism places greater merit on *motivations* than on passions.

By one Hindu authority, the cloning research itself is in violation of *ahiṁsā*. "Several of Wilmut's sheep were killed and autopsied by the researchers after their fetuses died. In *Āyurveda*, research on animals is allowed only to benefit the animal." A common mistake is repeated here, especially by those who would incorporate Āyurveda into a pure system of vegetarianism. The fact is that Caraka has copious recipes for dishes made of birds and animals for consumption by people in weakened conditions. There is indeed the taking of life, but when this is directed toward the goal of human welfare, it is morally justified. Failure to do so would incur the violation of *ahiṁsā*.

Tiruchi Mahaswamigal (founder of Kailash Ashram, India), points out that cloning "is not new to our cultural history. . . . We did not call it cloning, but there were other methods of procreation. Presently we do not require any such alternative methods of procreation for population, so man need not develop them." The point that is missed in this response is that cloning is not intended as an alternate method "of procreation for population"; its basic purpose is therapeutic, designed for the eradication of disease.

Paramhans Swami Maheswarananda (Founder, Sri Deep Madhvananda Ashram, Europe/India) opposes cloning, because it is "contrary to ethical and moral principles." He quotes Master Bhagwan Sri Deep Narayan Mahaprabhu: "Do not go against the nature, or else it will take revenge, and you will have to suffer the consequences." The principle of not going contrary to nature stands firm as a general principle, but with reference to cloning it is imprecise. The truth is that Mother Natutre herself has been in the business of cloning in the production of identical twins. There is more fact than fiction that the Ashwins, twin physicians to the gods, were clones of each other!

More serious problems are raised by Swamis Omkarananda Saraswati (Founder, Omkarananda Ashram, Europe/India) and Chidanand Saraswati (Head, Parmath Niketan, India). The first bemoans the folly of producing "unfortunate artificial copies of human beings," and the second believes "it would be unfortunate if all persons looked like one another; God intends a rich variety." The fears of the swamis are valid. Āyurveda insists: human individuality must be preserved at all times. However, as in the production of twins, nature itself is involved in cloning, with no dire results. This is because a duplicate body does not make a duplicate person. Whether produced naturally or artificially, clones are identical only physically. Identical twins become different individuals in the process of growing up. Environmental influences and personal choices make them different. The clone's brain would be far different from that of the donor, as it must start from scratch and build its own world of experiences. A cloned Mahatama Gandhi, for example, might turn out to be a serial killer, or a cloned Einstein could become a moron.

The facts are: identical genes do not produce identical people, as we all know with identical twins. In fact, twins are more alike than clones would be, since they have at least shared the uterine environment, and are usually raised in the same family. Parents could clone a second child who eerily resembled their first in appearance, but all of the evidence suggests the two would have very different personalities.

From the perspective of karma, which is the locus of individuality in Hinduism, the doctrine points to a clone building up his or her own personality by interaction of its peculiar *saṁskāras* (memory traces) and *vāsanas* (habit patterns), as spelled out in Patañjali's *Yoga Sūtras*.

In addition to the creation of personality differences as a consequence of diverse life experiences, the spectre of "Xerox Copies" is ruled out because age is also a factor for differentiation, as in the case of Dolly.

Having distinguished our line of thought from some traditional views discussed in *Hinduism Today*, we now present our views of Hindu bioethics on human cloning.

Two positions emerge in the above discussion: To Clone? or Not to Clone? One is a *prohibitive* stance, the other, a *permissive* stance. Hindu bioethics stands somewhere between the two.

Hindu bioethics enters the discussion on cloning, guided by three principles:

- Nonmaleficence
- Beneficence
- Autonomy

The principle of *nonmaleficence* is derived from *ahiṁsā* (noninjury). Its object of concern is the safety of fetuses and/or potential children whose well-being must not be sacrificed on some high altar of promoting a greater social and scientific good. Any procedure that places children at undue risk is morally problematic. Wilmut himself is opposed to cloning human beings at this stage of its technological development, because researchers would have to reckon with high failure rates. Scientists at the Univesity of Hawaii concur—risks would be substantial. Of 274 tries at cloning Fibro, the male mouse, using cells from a tail, all but three fetuses died. And two of the three survivors died within an hour of birth, according to an article by Wakayama and Yanagimachi in the journal *Nature Science* (June, 1998).

Therefore, in the interests of nonmaleficence, Hindu bioethics concludes that it is morally unacceptable for any scientific agency to attempt to create a child using somatic cell nuclear transfer cloning, because the current scientific evidence makes it clear that this technique is not safe for humans. Accordingly, it is in favor of the National Bioethics Advisory Commission's recommendaton to maintain a moratorium on the use of federal funds for human cloning, and that the private sector voluntarily follow suit.

At the same time, Hindu bioethics is on the side of a "sunset" provision in any federal legislation, whereby an impartial, qualified body of supervisors will be assigned the task of reviewing the situation with safety interests, prior to the expiration of the moratorium. To the extent that the needs for safety are satisfied, a window could then be opened in which the public is given the opportunity to debate the ethical and social issues spawned by the possibility of human cloning.

Next, Hindu bioethics turns to the principle of *beneficence*. The *vaidya* is exhorted in the medical *saṃhitās* always to keep the welfare of the patient first and foremost. In the event that the concerns of nonmaleficence are appropriately satisfied, and safety issues are adequately met, one could consider selective cases in which human cloning could be right, such as the victim of an acute form of leukemia who desperately needs a compatible source of bone marrow. We have already seen this scenario played out in the case of the couple that had a child to save their teenage daughter. A futuristic scenario may be thus: A baby girl is born free of the gene that causes Tay-Sachs disease, even though both of her parents are carriers. The reason? In the embryonic cell from which she was cloned, the flawed gene was replaced with normal DNA.

The mere mention of any such cases is bound to raise an alarming hew and cry, but when you are at the receiving end, when you are the person needing that bone marrow, the technology is welcomed as a blessing in disguise. Notwithstanding the soundness of Mrs. Ullal's (earlier) objection that a child should be begotten in passion, not made, one could point to the record numbers of children brought into the world through the comparable case of in vitro fertilization. All of these babies were *made, not begotten*. Yet there is no evidence of complaints that their mode of birth makes them feel like *products* rather than *persons*. None has been heard to say, "I'm only a test tube baby; I had the bad fortune of coming into the world without the benefit of the loving sexual embrace of my parents." In the absence of technology, they would not have the beneficent gift of life.

What is also missed in the conservative analysis of this procedure is that cloning is challenged as a *substitute* to nature's way of bringing a child into the world, instead of as a *alternate way*, necesitated by circumstances. It is this sensitivity to cirumstance that makes Hindu bioethics opposed to branding human cloning as *intrinsically wrong*. The genius of Hindu ethics is that it allows for a *dharma in extremis*. Its strength is autoplasticity.

The stance that human cloning is intrinsically wrong, under any conceivable circusmstances, underestimates the power of human ingenuity and its beneficent effects. The greatest benefits of cloning research are tied to the greatest medical problems we face today. Both cancer and the aging process involve genetic changes at the cellular level. Thus a better understanding of how genes work might someday have beneficent implications for anti-cancer and anti-aging treatments.

In addition to the principles of *nonmaleficence* and *beneficence*, Hindu bioethics is also committed to the principle of *autonomy*. Patañjali's karma doctrine affirms that we are all free agents. In the context of right priorities, autonomy has an important place. The principle of autonomy provides the basis for procreative or reproductive rights, including the right of self-replication. Hindu bioethics upholds the principle of autonomy out of respect for human individuality, provided its exercise inflicts no harm to the children reproduced. However, since there is no assurance of the safety factor at this time in cloning procedures, Hindu bioethics steers clear of any permissive policy that is based *solely* on autonomy. Thus in Hindu ethics *the principle of autonomy is regulated by the principles of beneficence and nonmaleficence*, and when the needs of the latter two are not met, autonomy steps back. In Hindu terms, *ahiṁsā* being the highest virtue, must be given precedence over other values.

Finally, we address the question of "Playing God," which not only appears in the title of the piece in *Hinduism Today*, but in more subtle forms in each of the sections we have devoted to genetics—*The Human Genome Project, Genetic Engineering*, and *Cloning*. All mythologies aside: What is the position of Hindu bioethics on this bedrock theme? Should Hindus support it or oppose it? We already know the answers of Hinduism's most prominent leaders—*Oppose*!

Āyurveda's rational orientation invites us to think through this tricky terrain, step by step.

Step One: Suffering is a fact of life. This is the "First Noble Truth" of Buddhism, but is present in all Indian analyses of the human condition. Recent scientific discoveries of widespread genetic defects is proof that whatever be the perfect will of God for us humans, biological perfection is not one of them. *Life is dukkha*.

Step Two: A basic goal of medicine should be the amelioration of suffering. As a motivation, this is the noblest of all human aspirations.

Step Three: The science of genetics is a powerful way to remove suffering.

Step Four: The prime motivation of the science of genetics is to alleviate suffering. In the words of Francis Collins, director of the National Human Genome Research Institute: "The primary reason we are doing the genome project, the primary reason why there is such a focus on genetics in medical research right now, is the desire to harness this new approach to better understand and treat disease."[4]

Step Five: Accepting the premise that the science of genetics is the most efficient way to accomplish the goal of mitigating suffering, and that its prime motivation is to do so, it follows that it would be the most *adharmic* position for a rational person to say we should not be pursuing genetic research because it might get misused. This is not a blank cheque. Projects are as good or as bad as the people who run them. But we would be guilty of *hiṁsā* if we block human ingenuity, considering its ability to heal and restore countless million sufferers. The "long life" Āyurveda promotes would not be so long, were it not for the most promising discoveries of those times. Swami Chidanand Saraswati captures the innovative spirit of Caraka, including his warnings against the medical quackery of his day. The swami says: "A lot of evil can result from human cloning [and genetic engineering, in general]. However the extension of knowledge should not be stopped. Genetic engineering should go on under strict conditions of global regulation with input from the different nations, races and genders."[5]

CHAPTER 12

THE ETHICS OF POPULATION GROWTH

> Every ten seconds the world's population increases by 27 people. . . . With luck those 27 people will have enough food to eat and clean water to drink and will dwell in decent homes. They will become farmers, teachers, salespeople, and magazine editors. If all goes well, they will live to a ripe old age.
>
> They will also clear forests for agriculture and housing, generate bargefuls of sewage, and choke rivers with fertilizer runoff. And therein lies the challenge of balancing world population growth with our planet's biodiversity.
>
> —Editorial, *National Geographic,* October 1998

Explosive human growth was one of the defining characteristics of the twentieth century. Global population quadrupled—growing faster than at any time in history. At the beginning of the twentieth century, the world's population was approximately 1.5 billion; at the end, it had reached 6 billion on the symbolic date of October 12, 1999. Notwithstanding improved methods of contraception and family planning, 7 billion may be reached in shorter order.

The Population Reference Bureau (PRB), based in Washington, DC, ascribes this potentially unprecedented human growth to the age and structure of the population.

The PRB report (1999) states, "Past levels of high fertility have resulted in many children—record high numbers in the youngest ages. . . . When all of those children reach childbearing age, even if they have fewer children than previous generations, population will still contine to grow; total births will continue to exceed total deaths as these youth become parents."[1]

According to the State of World Population 1999 report by the United Nations Population Fund, how fast the next billion people are added, the effect on natural resources, on the environment, and on the quality of life, will depend on policy and funding decisions taken in the next five to ten years.[2]

Hence, though the rate of population growth is decelerating, the world's population increases by 80 million every year. Half of all of these people are under twenty-five years of age.

By the year 2050, the United Nations predicts the world population will rise to 8.9 billion.[3] More than 95 percent of that growth will be in the developing countries of Africa, Latin America, and South Asia, which are already struggling to accommodate their current populations. The more developed countries are projected to double their numbers in 264 years, the less developed in forty years or less.

All these statistics combine to set the most pressing agenda for the twenty-first century: *to achieve a balance between population growth, natural resources, and economic development, which are essential for the improvement of the quality of life for all.*

A major player in these matters is India, which, as of May 1999, became a "billionaire" in population. From before the ancient Vedic period, it took thousands of years for India's population to reach the Himalayan heights of 1 billion; now it may take just 100 years to add another billion in this very century—an Everest upon an Everest! Of the twenty countries that account for 70 percent of world population, India is the highest—it contributes one-sixth of the world's population.[4]

Latest figures of the Population Reference Bureau (June 2000) predict that by 2050, India could surpass China as the most populous country on this planet. Of its 1 billion, 114 million are younger than age four—"a group that if counted on its own would amount to the llth largest country in the world."[5]

India's population increases by more than 30 a minute, 1,815 per hour, 1.3 million per month and 15.7 million, the equivalent of the Netherlands' population, per year.

During a trip to India (December 1999), Werner Fornos, president of the Population Institute, an NGO with seventy-two countries as its members, said that "India lacks political commitment to family planning." He felt that in a country where less than 3 percent of the budget is allocated to health care, family planning and population control programs will not be very successful.[6] Avabhai Wadia, founder of the Family Planning Association of India, agrees. In an interview (December 8, 1999) she said: "From ancient times India has had a large population and it was an asset—it helped in development. It is only now that it has taken a turn for the worse with poverty and illiteracy becoming so prominent." For the success of family planning programs, Wadia said awareness followed by action were the key.[7]

Hindu bioethics embraces the notion of family planning. It is discussed in great detail in the medical manuals of Āyurveda. Caraka believes that young couples should be fully educated about questions of fertility and pregnancy. A baby should not be born as a result of ignorance in respect to sexual activity, and should not arrive unwanted. A "love child," in his book, is not the offspring of unwed passion, but a gift of life that is planned in most meticulous fashion. You do not just jump into bed. A family is too important to be without planning. It begins with the fitness of the man and woman, which recognizes genetic responsibility; is carried over into sex selection, with equality toward both sexes; and then orchestrates sexual positions with erotic love. In his chapter on "Principles of Procreation," Caraka expounds the following:

> Now (I) shall mention the procedure by which the man and woman having undamaged sperm (in the case of the former) ovum and uterus (in the case of the latter) and desirous of excellent progeny can achieve that object.
>
> First of all both man and woman should undergo unction and fomentation and thereafter purify themselves by emesis and purgation so that they come gradually to normalcy. . . .
>
> After the onset of menstruation, for three days and nights, the woman should observe celibacy. . . . On the fourth day, she should be anointed and bathed from head and provided with white apparel along with the man. Now both the partners wearing white apparel and garland, with pleasant disposition and loving each other should enter into sexual intercourse on even days after bath if they desire male child or on odd days if they desire female child.
>
> One should not perform coitus with the female partner in her bending down or side position. . . . She should receive the seed (semen) while in supine position because in that condition *doṣas* remain in their normal position. . . . The woman subjected to over-eating, hunger, thirst, fear, detraction, grief, anger or having desire for other man or excessive coitus does not conceive or gives birth to abnormal child. One should avoid the woman too young, too old, suffering from prolonged illness or afflicted with any other disorder. These very defects are also in man. Hence man and woman should join together when they are free from all defects.
>
> When they are stimulated and are favourably disposed for coitus, they should go to the bed well-perfumed, well-covered and comfortable after taking favourite and wholesome food without over-eating, which the man should ascend with his right leg and the woman with the left one.[8]

Instructions continue, but the point is made that what happens in the family in terms of health, happiness, size, and quality is not left to God, to Nature, or to Chance but is the outcome of forethought and meticulous planning.

Thus, Hindu bioethics does not have to be sold on the merits of family planning; it is part of its moral mandate from early times. In a contemporary setting, its *principles* promote the cause of family planning, because:

- Family planning saves lives.
- Family planning prevents abortions.
- Family planning protects the environment.
- Family planning is what people want.

FAMILY PLANNING SAVES LIVES

According to USAID's International Population and Family Planning Assistance:

Throughout the developing world, millions of mothers and their children die each year due to complications from births that are too close together or too early or too late in a woman's life. Every day, more than 31,000 children under age five die—many from low birthweight or other pregnancy-related complications. And each year, more than 585,000 women die—at least one woman every minute of every day—of causes related to pregnancy and childbirth; 99% of those death are in developing countries.[9]

On the strength of its *preventive* orientation, the *principles* of Hindu bioethics promote family planning by:

- Preventing infant death through spacing births, at least two years apart
- Allowing women to delay motherhood
- Avoiding unwanted pregnancies and unsafe abortions
- Preventing the spread of HIV/AIDS and other STDs by providing condoms and other barrier methods

FAMILY PLANNING PREVENTS ABORTIONS

The World Heatlh Organization estimates that 40 percent of unintended pregnancies end in abortion. A minimum of 67,000 women die every year from the consequences of unsafe abortion. Hindu bioethics is opposed to the employment of abortion as a method of population control, either by individuals or by governments. Family planning could help couples prevent unintended pregnancies through use of effective modern methods of contraception.[10] Hindu bioethics takes a compassionate attitude of *dayā* toward the woman who has had an abortion, in place of harsh judgments that add guilt and misery to tragedy.

FAMILY PLANNING PROTECTS THE ENVIRONMENT

According to USAID, "More than 95% of population growth is occurring in the developing world, where population pressures are contributing to deforestation, water and food shortages, global warming, wildlife extinction and other environmental concerns."[11]

By slowing the growth of population, family planning helps reduce strain on the environment; eases pressures on fragile political and social systems; and reduces the impacts of unemployment, poverty, and cross-border migration.

FAMILY PLANNING IS WHAT PEOPLE WANT

The charge that family planning programs are imposed on poor nations and on poor women for economic, political, or social reasons is generally unfounded. Statistics show couples representing different countries, religions, and cultures do want smaller families than the actual size of families in their setting. "At least 12 million couples in the developing world still want to space or limit childbearing but do not have access to contraception, and the number of reproductive-age couples is expected to increase by at least 20 million a year."[12] China is about the only exception.

In addition to its adoption by couples, most governments recognize that family planning programs play an important role in human and eco nomic development and are eager to give it support.

Summing up the position of Hindu bioethics on population control, it is clear that its principles of *prevention* and *procreation* provide grist for the movement of two cycles: one (a) *adharmic* (vicious), and one (b) *dharmic* (virtuous).

(a) In the *adharmic cycle*, when families fail to plan, and where love is imbalanced by a preoccupation with passion, women become sick, because mothers have births that are too early, too late, or too closely spaced. Sick women have sicker children. And higher infant mortality leads to more births, as women calculate they must have many babies to beat the odds. It all adds up to a vicious cycle. This is *adharma*.

(b) In the *dharmic* cycle, where family planning is practiced, and where enlightened love is the basis of passion, women are healthier because they prevent births that are too early, late, or closely spaced. Healthy mothers produce healthy children. And because of low infant mortality, women do not feel the need to have many children as insurance against the survival of a few. This makes for a virtuous cycle. *This is dharma*.

In addition to family planning as a means to slowing population growth, Hindu bioethics also promotes other avenues, such as the improvement of women's education and socioeconomic status; increasing child survival; and reducing poverty. All these points are connected and must be dealt with as parts of a single package. This was the message of Dr. Karan Singh, then India's Minister of Health, at the Bucarest Conference on World Population (1994). He noted that for more than twenty years India had been trying to reduce fertility. He said, however, that family levels could be "effectively lowered only if family planning became an integral part of a broader strategy to deal with the problems of poverty and underdevelopment."[13]

Sunita Kishor, member of a Maryland-based research group (ORC Macro) that is making a survey of family health in India, states that though the Indian government has made slow but steady progress toward advancing literacy, educational levels differ from one region to another. Fornos has a similar observation. He is highly appreciative of Kerala, a southern state, which won the state award for slowest population growth. "You don't have to look at any other country for examples. Kerala is worthy of emulation with its 97 per cent literacy."[14] By the opposite token, in Uttarpradesh, a northern state, the illiteracy rate for females older than six is about 68 percent; the national rate is 57 percent.

If it were its own country, Uttarpradesh's 170 million people would make it the fifth largest, tieing with Brazil, and bigger than Pakistan (151 million).

Kishor remarks: "It's not just a population issue, but it's also the attitude toward girls. The culture doesn't promote the view that girls can go out and earn a living for themselves. If a parent has a daughter, they are really viewed as if you have to marry them off as quickly as possible."[15]

Thus a vicious triangle emerges, bounded by *gender, illiteracy,* and *fertility*. The Indian government talks about its commitment to empower people to have knowledge and the means to control their fertility, but that goal is not possible without the eradication of illiteracy among females. Fornos notes: "It is found that an eighth grade educated woman has half the number of children than her uneducated counterpart."[16] Current adult literacy rates stand at: female—39.4 percent; male—66.7 percent.[17]

Sunita Kishor's remarks that beyond the population problem lie negative attitudes toward the female gender is our cue to address two issues essential to a population ethic: *marriage* and *offspring*.

Traditional *Hindu marriage* has a fivefold purpose: pleasure *(rati)*, parenthood *(prajātī)*, companionship *(sakhya)*, sacrificial service *(yajña)*, and spiritual bliss *(ānanda)*. Due to the historic need for large families, it is underestandable how the primary meaning of marriage developed around the notion of *prajātī* (parenthood). This identification of marriage with procreation has tended to define the wife's role as biological. The young bride only becomes a fully fledged member of the husband's family when she produces a child, preferably a son. Without this, her traditional status has been in jeopardy. Today, with the need to limit the size of families, the social and spiritual purposes of marriage ought to be cultivated around the goal of *sakhya* or companionship. This sentiment is expressed in the words of the groom to the bride in the marriage hymn of the Ṛg Veda, "I take thy hand in mine, for happy fortune that thou mayest reach old age with me thy husband."[18]

Finally, in developing a population ethic, Hindus are obligated to face honestly the issue of equality of *offspring*. Prejudice and injustice run deep. They are hallowed by religion and flourish in a culture that is patriarchal to the core. Success in this area could not only mean a moral victory but reduction of the birth rate by a substantial percentage.

The need for a new philosophic perspective grows out of Hinduism's traditional preference for male offspring. The religious basis for this preference is the belief that the son rescues the souls of departed ancestors from hell. Manu says:

> By a son one conquers the worlds, by a son's son one attains the infinite, by the son of a son's son one attains the region of the sun. Since a son succours his father from the hell called *Put*; hence, the self-begotten one (Brahmā) has called a son, *Putra* (lit., deliverer from the hell of *Put*).[19]

The status of the eldest son in the Hindu family is unique. He has the right to offer the funeral cake *(piṇḍa)* at the time of the *śrāddha* ceremony marking the anniversary of the death of the father and ancestors.

Responsibility for performance of rites for the forefathers stems from the notion that the sins of commission and omission done by parents are visited upon their children. Retribution can be averted by means of the *śrāddha* rites. These household ceremonies are conducted every month for one year after the death. During this time it is believed that the deceased father moves in the air, not having been admitted to the company of the forefathers. At the conclusion of the year, a ceremony is performed by which the deceased is admitted to the assembly of the forefathers and thereby becomes a *pitri.*

Manu states that the firstborn son on whom the father passes his debt *(riṇam)* and by whom he gains immortality *(anantyam) i*s the only child begotten for the sake of *dharma (sa eva dharmajah putrah); a*ll others are the fruit of passion *(kāmajah).*[20]

The importance of the *śrāddha* rites elevates the role and status of the son and correspondingly devalues the daughter. When the dowry, which the father must give upon the marriage of the daughter, is also calculated, her liability increases as compared with a son, who is an asset to his father in every way—spiritual, social, and economic. No wonder there are always accounts of female infanticide, especially among low-caste families.

It is time that Hindus reevaluated the unethical accretions that have grown around their eschatology. Hindu beliefs are held on progressive levels of sophistication, but *śrāddha,* though philosophically low, is not recognized as low, because it caters to a host of nonreligious factors that assume male superiority and are difficult to eject in a patriarchal culture.

Philosophically viewed, the declared function of a son "as an instrument for cleansing his ancestors in the funeral rites" is purely magical. The private performance of *śrāddha,* out of the sight of eunuchs, outcastes, heretics, or pregnant women, for fear that it might be rendered "unclean," is both magical and superstitious. It demeans Hindu ethics to be associated with beliefs about collective guilt, about doing good deeds to acquire merit, and about the notion that offerings (excluding "unconsecrated grain of lentils, gourds, garlic, onions, or red vegetable extracts," and salt) somehow nourish the ethereal bodies of the departed ancestors, enabling them to perform works of merit that will advance them toward their goal of union with *Brahman.*[21]

Hindu eschatology is more rationally served by the philosophic belief in karma, which asserts that each person makes his or her own heaven and hell. Moreover, our deeds are personal and private and therefore cannot accrue for good or for ill to other persons, aside from the natural impact of socially conditioned forces. Most important, a religion that views life as unitive is ethically inconsistent when it elevates the salvific value of one sex over the other. It is strange that a religion that establishes the worship of animals should discriminate against its own daughters. In today's world of exploding populations, Hindu bioethics holds there is a more ethical way to affirm the continuity between the generations and to honor and immortalize the names of beloved ancestors. Such *dharma* is performed by intelligent planning of the family, by postponing childbearing, by educating women, by getting men to assume reproductive responsibility, and by enhancing gender equality, equity, and empowerment of women. By so doing, we can promote a *smaller world* by promoting a more *just world*.

CHAPTER 13

THE ETHICS OF AGING
Maximizing the Quality of Later Life

America is aging. Since the 1960s, we have shifted from "the greening of America" to "the graying of America." According to figures from the Kennedy Institute of Ethics, "Persons 65 years of age and over made up 9.2% of the population in 1960 and 12.3% in 1990; this figure is projected to increase to 20% by 2020 as the baby boom generation becomes 65 (11, Sonnefeld 1991). Within this group, the percentage of those over 85 years of age. . . will double from 3 million in 1990 to 6.1 million in 2010 (11, Samuelson 1992)."[1] The benchmark age of sixty-five has an interesting if somewhat ironic origin. A half-century ago, when Congress was debating Social Security legislation, it asked the Library of Congress to research an appropriate age for payments to begin.

A study revealed that in the 1880s, when Bismarck was chancellor of Germany, he had established a rather primitive social security system that benefited people if and when they reached sixty-five.

Although people were living longer in the 1930s than in the 1880s, Congress picked up on that figure sixty-five. It became embedded in our culture as the dividing point between middle and old age. Today those sixty-five can anticipate living another sixteen or more years. What factors are responsible for these demographic trends toward longevity?

On the objective side, experts point out that "the low birth rate in the U.S. in the last several years has influenced the proportion of the population 65 and over more than anything else."[2] Another major factor is "decreasing mortality, due in large part to the availability of high technology within acute-care settings."[3] If there is a secret to long life, it is surely in the genes. Temperament, also genetically mediated, may play a role in longevity, too.

On the subjective side, it is of interest to note that lifestyle, the bedrock of Āyurvedic medicine and the nursery of Hindu bioethics, is also a contributor to longevity. Lifestyle involves cultivating close companions; maintaining a network of social support; having the knack to manage stress; wisdom to accept losses and make adjustments; refusal to quit; keeping physically fit; keeping mentally alert; being spiritually grounded.

Today foremost in the quest for longevity are the molecular biologists. With awesome speed they are "teasing apart" the hormonal, cellular, and genetic underpinnings of old age.[4] However, in their promising assault on the biology of aging they are stirring up some difficult ethical questions:

- How do we now define old age?
- What are the markers of age? What should they be?
- Are longer lives necessarily better lives?
- Who should decide how long a person should live?
- How would future generations fare in a world where the elderly—no matter how beloved—refused to depart?[5]

The ethical question we focus upon is one we believe is uppermost in the minds and hearts of people everywhere, namely: *How can we age well?*

MODELS OF AGING

In the current literature, we can identify the emergence of three distinct models of aging in the United States. We call them:

1. The Social Model
2. The Medical Model
3. The Success Model

The Social Model

Over the past twenty years, gerontologists, humanists, health professionals, social workers, and organized elders have waged a campaign against the "myths" of old age, and have sought to replace negative images of aging with positive ones. The target of their attack is the notion of "ageism," understood as a systematic scheme to stereotype and discriminate against older people, much on the order of racism and sexism.

The term "ageism" was coined by psychiatrist Robert Butler, in 1968. Through his positions as director of the National Institute on Aging (1974–1982) and head of the department of geriatrics and adult development at Mt. Sinai Hospital, New York, Butler has been an ardent foe of prejudice and age discrimination. His Pulitzer Prize-winning book *Why Survive?* (1975) is still the best-known expose of aging in America. He describes ageism as having deep social roots, expressed in "stereotypes and myths, outright disdain and dislike, or simply subtle avoidance of contact; discriminatory practices in housing, employment and services of all kinds; epithets, cartoons and jokes." Such stereotyping provides members of society with justification to ignore the plight of the old, and also to disengage themselves from having to face the facts of their own aging and death.

The social approach to aging attends less to the prolongation of life as to the improvement of its quality, especially the quality of what used to be known as the declining years. "Resisting the equation of old age with loss of powers, proponents of this approach demand a more active social role for those who, though past middle age, have by no means outlived their usefulness."[6] These humanitarians demonstrate that old age is a "social" rather than a "biological" category. In their view "the modern problem of old age . . . originates less in physical decline than in society's intolerance of old people, its refusal to make use of their accumulated wisdom, and its attempt to relegate them to the margins of social existence."[7]

Thus by debunking the myths of old age, the social model stands out for its vision of hope for the elderly; for its recognition of the special contributions seniors have to make toward the social good; for its critique of a culture that equates seniority with senility; and for its refusal to allow the elderly to go gently into the night.

The Medical Model

Two books that best represent this perspective are: *Prolongevity* by Albert Rosenfeld, and *No More Dying: The Conquest of Aging and the Extension of Human Life* by Joel Kurtzman and Phillip Gordon.[8] For these authors, old age is a "medical problem" that medical science is equipped to eliminate in the twenty-first century.

According to Rosenfeld, the elderly should consult their doctors for the problems of old age. He attributes the extension of the life span to modern medicine; he anticipates that by the year 2025 "most of the major mysteries of the aging process will have been solved"; and with great optimism he predicts "we will soon have in our hands the biological tools to bring about . . . the long-sought elixir of life, in one form or the other."[9]

The good news according to Albert Rosenfeld is that we are on the brink of "eradicating old age."

With similar optimism, Kurtzman and Gordon predict that living to the age of a hundred and fifty is now within scientific reach, by means of progress in genetics; by transplant technology; and by the simulation of organic processes through research in bionics. Other scientists, representing prestigious institutions, join their voices to this hopeful chorus. Alex Comfort proclaims: "If the scientific and medical resources of the United States alone were mobilized, aging could be conquered within a decade." Augustus Kinzel, former president of the Salk Institute, is confident that "we will lick the problem of aging completely, so that accidents will be essentially the only causes of death." Robert Sinsheimer, Cal Tech, is equally optimistic "we know of no intrinsic limits to the life span. How long would you like to live?"[10]

To set these predictions in perspective, it should be pointed out that each one of these projections comes with a price tag attached, along with the caveat that the medical goals can only be reached if they are backed up by enormous resources required to conquer a specific disease being targeted by the agency.

The Success Model

Successful Aging by John W. Rowe, M.D., and Robert Kahn, Ph.D., is a product of the MacArthur Foundation Study of Successful Aging. The ten-million dollar project took several forms, including "studies of over a thousand high-functioning older people for eight years, to determine the factors that predict successful physical and mental aging; detailed studies of hundreds of pairs of Swedish twins to determine the genetic and lifestyle contributions to aging; laboratory-based studies of the response of older persons to stress; and nearly a dozen studies of brain aging in humans and animals."[11]

The book itself deals with three basic questions about human aging:

1. What does it mean to age successfully?
2. What can each of us do to be successful at this most important life task?

3. What changes in American society will enable more men and women to age successfully?

The context in which the MacArthur Study was born is illuminating. Throughout the 1970s and early 1980s, interest in gerontology and geriatrics was driven by a knowledge of the social, economic, and health care consequences of the graying of Americans. "Despite this energy, the progress of gerontology began to stall in the mid-1980s. Lacking was the conceptual foundation required to understand aging in all its aspects—biological, psychological, and social. There was a persistent preoccupation with disability, disease, and chronological age, rather than with the positive aspects of aging."[12]

In the definition of the authors, successful aging is the ability to "maintain three key behaviors or characteristics":

1. Low risk of disease and disease-related disability
2. High mental and physical function
3. Active engagement with life[13]

On the matter of *avoiding disease,* Rowe and Kahn say that modern medicine has developed as an applied science of "repair rather than prevention," and that even though it is becoming more inclusive, "the field of geriatrics has been slower to make this shift."[14]

On maintaining *mental and physical function,* the authors say that older people want to be independent and the MacArthur research has three reassuring messages for them: (1) many of the fears about functional loss are exaggerated; (2) much functional loss can be prevented; and (3) many functional losses can be regained.[15]

On continuing *engagement with life,* MacArthur research shows something relatively new, that our "happy activities" are essential to successful aging.

> Thirty years ago, something called "disengagement theory" was influential among gerontologists. This theory defined the main task of old age as letting go. The argument was that old age was a time at which people were required to give up their jobs, could no longer take part in the more strenuous forms of recreation, and sadly, had to say farewell to many old friends and family members. The final act of relinquishment was letting go of life itself.[16]

In summary the authors say: "We were trying to pinpoint the many factors that conspire to put one octogenarian on cross-country skis and another in a wheel-chair."[17]

CRITIQUE OF THE SOCIAL AND MEDICAL MODELS OF AGING

Here we wish to make a few critical comments on the social and medical models of aging, informed by Hindu ethical principles. This will be followed by our discussion of the Hindu model, with special reference to the model of "Successful Aging."

Though the social and medical approaches to aging are distinct and divergent, they do converge at certain critical points. We list these points of convergence as follows:

- A powerful aversion to the prospect of bodily decay
- A mutual understanding of old age and death as an imposition on the human race that is no longer acceptable
- A loathing for the image of life as a "brief candle"
- A fear of "losing our powers," being "left alone," and being handed over to "indifferent nurses"

What are the bases for these fears that make of old age a problem for proponents of the social and medical models?

First, *old age is seen as the harbinger of death*, and though fears of old age and death are normal, these ancient fears are intensified because we live in a materialistic society that has deprived itself of religion and shows little interest in posterity.[18]

Second, old age is not only seen as "the beginning of death," *the role and status of the elderly have depreciated in modern times*. Judged by the dominant cult of youth, the elderly are defined as useless and are treated as superflous. Productivity is defined in terms of physical strength, good looks, charisma, skill, innovation, and adaptability, whereas experience and wisdom are reckoned too elusive for the computer age.

The elderly are not only neglected; *they are abused*. An estimated one million elderly people were abused in 1996, according to a report by the National Center on Elder Abuse.[19] That figure is up from the 1991 estimate of 735,000.

As more Americans live past age sixty-five, longevity is carrying a sobering cost. Reports of domestic abuse against the elderly increased 150 percent from 1986 to 1996—from 117,000 cases to 293,000. Hundreds of thousands more go unreported, because a relative is the abuser and the elderly person is reluctant to say anything. Often, they are dependent on that person who is abusing them to take care of them. It is fear of not knowing what will be next if they are taken out of that person's care.

Greed and abuse are often intertwined, with the physical abuse being the symptom and the financial abuse being the motivation.

Additionally, stress of caring for aging parents can sometimes lead to abuse, as can unresolved tensions between children and parents that build up over a lifetime.

Medicine also mistreats the elderly.[20] Hamstrung by biases and limited facts, doctors routinely deliver shoddy care to old people. Many old people do not get the screening tests they should; doctors tend to overload elderly people with unnecessary pills, or, conversely, fail to prescribe needed medications; surgeons either rush old patient into futile or harmful surgery or throw in the towel prematurely; for numerous lab tests commonly ordered on elderly people, "normal" results remain undefined, making it hard to separate symptoms of disease from signs of old age.

Much of this mistreatment starts with training. At a time when the elderly population is shooting upward, only eight of the nations's 126 medical schools require separate courses in geriatric medicine. And it is only recently that the "elderly are being included in research trials, which doctors rely on to formulate treatment plans. A high proportion of published heart-drug studies, for example, exclude anyone over 75, the very people who most risk dying of heart disease."[21]

Society expects older people to be sedentary, and many expect it of themselves. According to a Harvard publication: "Only 10% of Americans over 65 jog, play tennis, cross-country ski or engage in other vigorous exercise on a regular basis. Meanwhile, the inactive majority lose about 30% of their muscle mass between 20 and 70."[21]

Third, in addition to objective sociological and biological factors, old age is a problem because of *psychological causes*. This represents the subjective side of the problem. Too often analysts stop with an examination of objective experiences, but fail to uncover subjective experiences. Lasch says:

> If our era has a special dread of old age and death, this dread must arise out of some inner predisposition. It must reflect not only objective changes in

> the social position of the elderly but subjective experiences that make the prospect of old age intolerable.[22]

From one angle, it is perfectly rational to entertain fears of old age; from another angle it is irrational when people panic *prematurely*. The so-called midlife crisis starts with one's fortieth birthday, which is reckoned as the beginning of the end. *The midlife crisis is not for midlife anymore*. Thus, even the joys of the prime of life are eclipsed by what we see as the writing on the wall.

This *irrational fear* of old age and death is a cultural construct and is related to the dominance of the narcissistic personality in Western society. I call it the 'Old Mother Hubbard' syndrome. She is the lady who went to the cupboard, only to find that it was bare. Similarly the narcissistic person takes an inventory of his or her inner resources and discovers there is precious little. This person therefore "looks to others to validate his sense of self." He has a compelling need to be admired for his macho looks, celebrity, or power—all attributes that are affected by the march of time. "Unable to achieve satisfying sublimations in the form of love and work, he finds that he has little to sustain him when youth passes him by."[23] The narcissistic person takes no interest in the future and does little to provide him or herself with the traditional consolations of old age, namely faith in the transcendent and the belief that future generations will in some sense carry on the tasks of the older.

THE HINDU MODEL OF AGING

> When a householder sees his skin wrinkled and his hair white and the sons of his sons, then he may resort to the forest. . . . Let him always be industrious in reciting the Veda. . . . In summer, let him expose himself to the heat of five fires, during the rainy season live under the open sky, and in winter be dressed in wet clothes, thus gradually increasing the rigour of his austerities. . . . Then after abandoning all attachment to world objects. . . let him always wander alone, without any companion, in order to attain final liberation.[24]

A prima facie reading of this passage presents the Hindu view as a radically alternative vision to the social and medical models, and particularly to the model of "Successful Aging." From the Western point of view, the Hindu model is a brief for *unsuccessful aging*. In the words of one reviewer, "To head off to the forest when your hair turns white and you become a grandparent—and there, expose yourself to brutal summer heat and in winter to don wet clothes—this would do little to safeguard health. Instead of seeking to be engaged with life, the Hindu strives for disengagement. Active engagement, according to Rowe and Kahn, involves participation in a social network and in productive work 'that creates goods and services of value.'"[24]

On closer examination, the Hindu model is in many regards *on common ground with the new paradigm of Rowe and Kahn.* The research of successful aging corroborates the fundamental thesis of Āyurveda that *in terms of life's determinants, lifestyle need not be sacrificed to genes.* The book points out that there is increasing evidence that the rate of physical aging is not, as was once believed, determined by genes alone, and that lifestyle factors have powerful influences as well. Additionally, in terms of the first two counts of the book's definition of successful aging there is considerable agreement, but the Hindu model parts ways on the third count.

Basically, points one and two of the MacArthur study cover the need for high levels of *physical and mental functioning.*

Physically, the Hindu renunciate who takes to the forest has gray hair and wrinkled skin, but these signs of wear and tear should not suggest decrepitude. In order to survive the rigors of life in the forest, he has to be at low risk of disease and disease-related disability. Flight from wild animals, climbing, carrying wood, fording streams and rivers are not feats for the faint of heart or weak of limb.Whether by contrivance or not, he must be equal to the demands made upon his body by the changing seasons, especially the monsoons, and by all of the physical challenges of his environment. He gets more than his share of exercise by wandering, mile upon mile. His motivation in exercise is to gradually increase the rigor of his austerities in the pursuit of detachment, but the physical effects of this spartan regimen are to burn up unhealthy fat, strengthen muscles, harden bones, improve the cardiovascular system, while partaking of a diet prepared by Mother Nature herself.

It is clear that the forests of ancient India were not designated retreats for "R&R" (rest and relaxation), and as rewards for life-long labors, but places of physical rigor to promote mental and spiritual concentration.

In addition to qualifying for the physical definition of "successful aging," the Hindu model of aging meets the *standards of mental functioning.* We know that memory is the most important factor of successful aging, and that the brain is a muscle, subject to the law that you either use it or lose it. It is therefore with interest that we read instructions given to the forest dweller: "Let him always be *industrious in reciting* the Veda" (italics supplied). This called for exceptional memory, considering the amount of Vedic material he had to recite. More broadly, his whole life was one of contemplation, involving high levels of mental processing. *Contemplation is activity, not passivity.* And even more broadly, interaction with his environment was a constant test of wits, calling on a store of memory with reference to healing herbs, edible fruits, and tortuous trails.

Data for the primacy of mental and physical fitness can additionally be garnered from yoga philosophy and from the teachings of the medical *saṃhitās* on *Rasāyana* therapeutics. We have discussed this earlier and need not repeat ourselves. However, worthy of mention is the fact that for hundreds of years for countless thousands, these regimens have indeed fulfilled the fantasies of *Cocoon*, without having to resort to drugs and human growth hormones to fight the ravages of growing old.

Thus there seems to be a broad consensus between the MacArthur Foundation's paradigm for "successful" aging and the Hindu model in respect to the physical and mental definitions (points 1 and 2). This is not to suggest that the Hindu elder goes into the forest, as if he is entering a gym to build up body and mind, but both of these are the side effects of his spiritual pursuit for *mokṣa* (analagous to the relation of yoga and health).

Differences arise on the third count, namely: "a continuing active engagement with life." For Rowe and Kahn, this means being part of some organization that gives you the outlet to be productively employed in the creation of "goods and services of value."

The sticking point is what is meant by "life." Kahn and Rowe have told us what they mean: living life successfully is to be *physically fit, mentally sharp, and socially engaged.* But the Hindu bioethicist asks: Are these the only criteria for evaluating the rewards of a long life? Certainly there is all this, but additionally there is something more to life. In the end, the forest dweller abandons all lesser rewards for one that is higher. "Age has granted him permission to cast off the myriad duties of midlife. By 'abandoning' all attachment to worldly objects, 'one is liberated to focus on life's truest goal—achieving union with God.'"[26]

That is, the Hindu model is based on the *primacy of the transcendent.* But in the bigger picture this goal must be seen as the progressive unfolding of values through separate stages of the human life cycle. These stages are known as *āśramadharma.*

Āśramadharma has several elements of gerontological significance, as Shrinivas Tilak has shown in his *Religion and Aging in the Indian Tradition.*[27]

First the *āśrama* model supplies an age-specific structure through which all of the diverse forms of human desires and aspirations are actualized in a timely manner. For instance, the student must not indulge in sexual pleasures, but must undergo rigorous discipline, not because sex is bad, but because, physically and mentally, the growing child must first learn the meanings of responsibility and self-control. Once he becomes a mature householder, the same young man is encouraged to give full expression to his sexual desires and social inclinations through raising a family. In addition, the householder is to pursue the delights of wealth within the bounds of moral law. Thus there is no denial of the claims of the body, once the body feels the need for sensate satisfaction.

With age, the biological clock begins to tick, as changes in the body diminish the intensity of carnal needs and set the stage for hungers that transcend the body. Thus in the progression of life, all *desires* and *aspirations* are valid and deserving of equal attention; and the mark of a full life is the extent to which a person allows a capacity to flourish when its time has come, and does not hanker after it when its time has gone. Each time is the best time, because it uniquely demarcates a different slice of life—*life that is ever new, even as it grows old.* Thus the wisdom to accept and adjust to all of the changes that life throws at us serves as the key to health and happiness. Conversely, most miseries of old age ensue from failure to adjust.

Second, this holistic view of the person, which recognizes a congery of human needs that are brought to fruition on successive levels of maturation, has a moral correlate. It states a person is *right* for a particular stage when he is *ripe* for that stage. Here ethics is identified, not only with philosophy and theology, but with biology and psychology. For the Hindu bioethicist, this cautions against a type of moralistic reasoning that passes judgments on the wants and wishes of the elderly, which is long on philosophy and theology but short on psychology and biology. The *principle of ripeness* should also help bioethicists understand some of the sudden decisions that old folks make, especially the decision that it is "time to go." It would be naively moralistic for young doctors, chaplains, and social workers to conclude that these elders are overcome by some suicidal urge, when actually they are tuned to an internal clock. To thwart the individuals's decision at this point could mean that conventional ideas of "*rightness*" have been allowed to block nature's rules of "*ripeness*."

Third, when the elder retires to the forest, it does not mean he is going into retirement. True, he is no longer active on the horizontal level, expressed through communitarian concerns; but when the concerns of the transcendent take a hold of him, activity shifts from the horizontal to the vertical level. This shift signifies the successive expansion of his mind from ego-consciousness, to family consciousness, world consciousness, and ultimately to Universal Consciousness, which is identification with total existence in its deepest being.

Often the last two stages of life spent in the forest are described as states of "disengagement," presumably because communitarian ties are cut off. But this image of the disengaged recluse in retirement is incorrect. It overlooks the fact that disengagement on the horizontal level is only the sign and signal for reengagement on the vertical level. The individual does not come to a stop; he is only shifting to a higher gear. Like a trapeze artist, he is "letting go" of one bar only to be catapulted to a higher bar. Life's most difficult tasks, requiring all of one's resources of body, mind, and spirit, are reserved for the last part of the journey. This projects an image of old age that is strenuous, optimistic, and full of joy. *Āśramadharma* nurtures faith in human dignity and human capacity, *not in spite of old age but because of old age.*

The Hindu model thus stands out as a paradigm of graceful aging. Because a person's skin has become wrinkled and his hair has turned white, and he no longer possesses the charm and vigor of his children and grandchildren, it does not mean his life is divested of value, that he has nothing more to live for, that life has passed him by. Hinduism says that people have value, not because they are youthful, in the pink of health, economically productive, and socially engaged, but because they have a hunger for the transcendent, which is the only known force whereby people can positively come to terms with their own mortality and maximize the quality of later life.

The impression should not be conveyed that the Hindu paradigm of aging is prescriptive. That would conflict with the inclusivistic impulse of this tradition. It accepts different paths to wholeness in different traditions. The contemplative quest, in or outside the forest, is not for everyone. The Hindu bioethicist therefore evaluates notions of 'good' or 'bad' as functional terms to characterize the route to wholeness that works best for an individual in life's second half.

CHAPTER 14

THE ETHICS OF DEATH AND DYING

Whence are we born? Whereby do we live, and whither do we go?
— Śvetāśvatara Upaniṣad

VIEWS OF DEATH

An Arabian proverb describes death as "a black camel, which kneels at the gates of all." Though death is a human universal, how people think about it, and the manner in which they cope with the losses that come with death, varies markedly from culture to culture. Anthropologist Sylvia Vatuk observes that "there are real differences between Indian and American ways of aging and death." In the 1970s she did research in a major Indian city, and reports her findings:

> Among these people I found attitudes toward aging and death that seemed much more positive than our own. There was a greater degree of acceptance of the inevitability of mortality, and more attention was given to preparing actively for the end of life. While the material circumstances of their lives were far less comfortable than our own, these people seemed better equipped, both cognitively and emotionally, to face the inevitability of aging, dying, and death.[1]

Vatuk acknowledges "it would be foolish to idealize or romanticize the situation of older people in India," suggesting that somehow they are "free from stress or that their deaths are free from fear, suffering, and pain." The terror of death is a universal human experience, and Indians are by no means exempt from its horrors; but differences in culture between Indians and Americans do make for differences in attitudes and methods of coping, as we shall see.

IMPLICATIONS FOR BIOETHICS

One aim of this chapter, and indeed the entire volume, is to highlight the need in American circles to consider the bioethics of death in cross-cultural perspective. Anthropological research makes a strong case for the fact that in addition to differences in the ethics of the termination of life among world cultures, "these differences in values and practices surrounding death in any society can be understood only within the context of that society's ecological and demographic situation, social system, and cultural beliefs."[2]

HINDU VIEWS OF DEATH

In his essay on Hindu perspectives of death, Anantanand Rambachan brings out with fine lucidity the diversity of views that have evolved over some 2,500 years, and are expressed in myths, rituals, religion, and philosophy.[3] We shall add to this store by introducing views of death found in the medical *saṃhitās*, generally overlooked by philosophers and theologians.

First we must dismiss the stereotype that Hindus are a "spiritual" people, who do not take this world seriously, and therefore are not afraid of death. The truth is quite opposite. Like all mortals, Hindus want to live like immortals. It should be clearly understood that Āyurveda did not invent the notion of longevity, because this quest is embedded in the entire Hindu ethos. We have witnessed this theme surface in the Vedic period, where prayers and sacrifices are offered for a life of "hundred autumns," the equivalent of immortality. The same goal of living to a hundred years is institutionalized in the later *āśramadharma* tradition of orthodox Brahmanism, in which each of the four cycles is set at twenty-five years. In later Hinduism, mythologies abound, telling stories of how aging and death are transformed, and youth restored, by means of listening to a powerful scripture, living in a holy place, attending to a saint, performing rituals, and practicing devotion. So there is no question of the value placed on *life in this world* by Hindus.

Parallel to the hope that old age and death can be reversed, the belief arises that humans are responsible for their own future existences, by virtue of their karma. This should not be construed as an attitude of fatalism, because 'fate' is not attributed to some external agency but is of one's own making.

From earliest times, philosophers and religious thinkers have conceived the fate of the deceased in several imaginative ways. We outline the main trends.

First, the Vedas introduce the *śrāddha* ritual, which is perpetuated into later Brahmanic-Hindu tradition. As part of funerary ceremonies, it affirms that death does not break the ties between the living and the dead, and that reciprocal relationships are possible after a family member has passed on. Offerings of water and funerary cakes *(piṇḍas)* are made to three immediate generations of the dearly departed's paternal and maternal forebears. With sustenance for their ethereal bodies, ancestors are enabled to gather merit that will hasten their progress through future births, until they achieve union with the divine. Family members who honor a deceased relative by the sincere and reverent performance of *śrāddha,* also accumulate merit.

Second, a more powerful belief in the early Vedic period that guaranteed postmortem survival was connected with *ṛta,* conceived as universal cosmic law. Persons who upheld the law in this life were assured the restoration of their physical bodies, social connections, and worldly enjoyments in a future life. By the same token, the Atharva Veda warns of suffering and torment in the afterlife for wrongdoers.

Third, during the Brāhmaṇas (ca. 950–700 B.C.), ritual action attained magical proportions. It was believed that through ritual intervention a sacrificer could fashion a body that he or she could occupy after death. Intimations of suffering in store for transgressors are also found.

Fourth, with the Upaniṣads (700–500 B.C.) we encounter a spirit that is quite different to that of the Brāhmaṇas. These philosophical and mystical texts present new insights into the nature of the person, and thus precipitate a paradigm shift.

Basically, the Upaniṣads distinguish between the essential self and the empirical self. The essential self, which is of the nature of existence-consciousness-bliss *(sat-chit-ānanda),* is at the core of each person's being. In reality it is one, but through the power of ignorance and desire for bodily attachment it assumes individuality that is constituted of body, mind, and intellect. The empirical self is then erroneously taken for the esssential self. As a result, the self or *ātman* becomes a prisoner in an ongoing cycle of death and rebirth. Though the round of transmigration has limited fulfillments through the achievement of superior births gained by ritual practice and moral action, *saṁsāra* is ultimately a hopeless process of suffering and dying, and therefore devoid of meaning.

> He . . . who has not understanding,
> Who is unmindful and ever impure,
> Reaches not the goal,
> But goes on to reincarnation *(saṁsāra)*.[4]

The empirical self to which the essential self is supposed to be attached undergoes changes in the world of the senses. It has three kinds of bodies: physical, subtle, and causal.

The physical body is the locus of all experience arising from the external world, and is the seat of consciousness in wakeful states. It is the product of the five elements (earth, water, fire, wind, space). In death, the body returns to its source. *Death only refers to the dissolution of the physical body.*

The second is the subtle body, so called because it is composed of seventeen elements that are finer than those of the physical body. These elements are: mind, intellect, five vital breaths (*prāṇa* in the heart; *apāna* in the anus; *samāna* in the navel; *udāna* in the throat; and *vyāna* suffusing the whole body); five organs of action (speech, hands, feet, anus, and the generative organ); and five organs of knowledge (ear, skin, eye, tongue, nose). Thus the subtle body is a composite coordination of a person's chief functions—vital, mental, and intellectual. The presence of the essential self, and its direct awareness, makes all of this to happen. Hence the subtle body is the *liṅga* or characteristic symbol of the proximity of the self.

The subtle body provides individual continuity and functions as the instrument of karma during the transmigration of the self from one body to the next. It conserves the moral consequences of a person's life, which then impact the direction of the person's rebirth. In terms of direct impact, karmic consequences fix the type of physical body and environment the person will inherit in his or her next birth; and in terms of indirect impact, moral consequences condition the individual's propensities for behavior. The Kaṭha Upaniṣad considers this objective connection between past and future an operation of nature itself: "Like a grain a mortal ripens! Like a grain he is born hither (a-jayate) again." When the subtle body disengages from the physical body, death ensues.

The actual process of disengagement is described in the Bṛhadāraṇyaka Upaniṣad as a "fading out." First the eye becomes united with the subtle body, and we say "He does not see"; next the nose, tongue, voice, ear, and mind get united, as the dying process continues its decline.

Finally, the intellect becomes united with the subtle body, and we say "He does not know."[5]

In light of the above, from a bioethical perspective it is important that doctors should be able to sense when the dying process has begun its course; should not attempt to foil the natural process through useless interventions and interruptions; and should let the patient die in peace.

At the same time, the patient's physical state should not obscure his or her state of spiritual consciousness. The body indeed influences the mind and the spirit, but the opposite is equally true. Therefore the individual must be kept as comfortable as possible, precisely in order to enable the spirit to have its final moments. The quality of one's state of consciousness at the terminus of life sets the stage for the exit of the subtle body from the physical body and also directs its future trajectory. The Gītā supports this theory with its claim that whatever is the focus of one's mind in the hour of death represents what one worships, and forms us in its image. "Whatever state of being he remembers, upon giving up his body at the end, to that he attains, O son of Kuntī; always being formed in that state."[6] The words "*sada tad bhava bhavitah*" convey the meaning of being permanently absorbed in the thought of something over an entire lifetime, which carries the seeds of its own future, and rules out any deathbed fancy.

The Kaṭha Upaniṣad describes the parting of the soul from the body with spectacular imagery:

> There are a hundred and one channels of the heart.
> One of these passes up to the crown of the head
> Going up by it, one goes to immortality.
> The others are for departing in various directions.[7]

This verse is borrowed from Chāndogya Upaniṣad (viii. 6.6.) where it is said that the soul of a man who has lived the pure life of a student of sacred knowledge *(brahmacarya)* and so "found the Self," will, at death, pass up a vein, known later as *suṣumṇā* (carotid vein), to an opening in the skull called the *brahmarandhram* or *vidṛti*. This refers to the aperture in the child's skull called the anterior fontanelle, by which, at the beginning of life, the soul first entered. From there the soul ascends by the sun's rays to the sun, which is a doorway to the Brahmā-world to those who know, but a transit place for nonknowers.

Life after death is envisioned in diverse forms in the Gītā and the Upaniṣads.

The Gītā declares: "The worshipers of the gods go to the gods; the worshipers of the ancestors go to the ancestors; sacrificers of the spirits go to the spirits; and those who sacrifice to Me come to Me."[8] Devotees who work their way up to the worlds of the gods, the ancestors and the spirits, are rewarded for their good works, but since these worlds are the objects of desire, and the fruits of human merit, once merit is depleted, individuals enter once more the cycle of *saṁsāra.*

The Upaniṣads entertain similar visions of future life in *svargaloka* and *brahmaloka.* The first is the world of heaven. It is earned by persons who have dedicated their lives to the public good; but since they do not possess liberating knowledge, they are not freed from the rounds of birth, death, and rebirth. The second is the world of the creator. Those who enter its portals do not return to *saṁsāra,* because they have a saving knowledge of *brahman,* albeit in anthropomorphic form. Further spiritual progress is assured, and with cosmic dissolution, these individuals achieve *mokṣa.*

Alongside these visions of heavenly worlds of pleasure for those who have lived righteous lives, there are descriptions of hell that await the unrighteous. In the Gītā Arjuna warns Kṛṣṇa that when lawlessness prevails, the women of the family are corrupted and this leads to the mixture of castes. "And this confusion brings the family itself to hell and those who have destroyed it; for their ancestors fall, deprived of their offerings of rice and water."[9] Hell is again mentioned as the just recompense for persons of demoniacal character, who "bewildered by many fancies, enveloped by the net of delusions and addicted to the satisfaction of desires . . . fall into an impure hell."

Descriptions of the diverse heavens and hells may be imaginary, but they do convey the scriptural principle of the rise and fall of the soul in accordance with karma. Descent into hell is not any more of a permanent state than ascent to a meritorious heaven.[10] Ultimately there is the hope that by passing through many forms of life, the individual soul will be given sufficient scope to find enlightenment and gain *mokṣa,* freed at last from the wheel of rebirth. The possibility of multiple rebirths and eventual release is an insight of Hinduism into the nature and destiny of man, which sets it apart from Christianity that believes "it is appointed unto men once to die, but after this the judgment" (Heb. 9.27).

The hope for *mokṣa* glimmers when death itself is seen from a different angle and serves as a paradigm for Release. This is because, as Reynolds observes, at the point of death, the soul experiences a fleeting moment of freedom from the material elements that hold it captive. He says:

> At this most profound level of Indian thought, death comes to serve as a prefiguration and model for various meditations and disciplines (classical yoga, devotional disciplines, tantra, etc.) through which the ties that bind man's self or soul to cosmic impermanence can be completely broken, and through which the ultimate soteriological goals of immortality and freedom can be finally definitively attained.[11]

This quest for immortality and freedom is classically expressed in the well-known prayer:

> From the unreal *(asat)* lead me to the real *(sat)*!
> From darkness lead me to light!
> From death lead me to immortality![12]

This prayer encapsulates the truth that unity with Brahman is the highest goal of human endeavor, for both this world and the next. Herein lies a person's ultimate value, greatest bliss, truest freedom, and deepest peace. Though exalted, perfect knowledge is possible in one's present life. Some say Brahmā-realization is only reached after death; but there is also the claim of *jīvanmukti* that liberation can be reached here and now. The Kaṭha Upaniṣad affirms: "When all the desires the heart harbours are gone, man becomes immortal and reaches Brahman here."[13]

Mokṣa is essentially experienced as freedom. It is freedom from self-centered individuality that attaches itself to the changing objects of the world, and therefore doomed to suffering. It is freedom from births and deaths, and hence transcends the limitations of time. It is freedom from the law of karma, leaving the released individual unaffected by good or bad deeds. It is freedom from ignorance that produces bondage. Freedom is not a condition that is created, but a reality that is recognized.

Several uplifting passages attempt to describe the state of *jīvanmukti*. The Muṇḍaka Upaniṣad brings out the experience of overcoming all distinctions of individuality ('name and form'), along with the rewards of soteriological knowledge.

> As the flowing rivers in the ocean
> Disappear, quitting name and form,
> So the knower, being liberated from name and form.
> Goes unto the Heavenly Person, higher than the high.

He, verily, who knows that supreme Brahmā, becomes very Brahmā. In his family no one ignorant of Brahmā arises. He crosses over sorrow. He crosses over sin *(papman)*. Liberated from the knots of the heart, he becomes immortal.[14]

IMPLICATIONS OF HINDU VIEWS ON DEATH AND DYING FOR BIOETHICS

On the basis of the sketch of Hindu philosophic views of death and dying we have just presented, we now draw out and capsulize elements that are important for doing bioethics.

- Death is the end of the body *(dehanta)*. It occurs with the dissolution of the subtle body from the physical body.
- Death is not the opposite of life. It is the opposite of birth.
- Death and life are markers on one continuous trajectory of life. They are not "different ontological entities in polar opposition to each other, but facets of a single, seemingly endless cycle."[15]
- Denial of the finality of death by affirming belief in the indestructible *ātman* reduces helplessness in the face of death.
- Karma connects a person with the past, present, and future dimensions of his or her life, and gives moral meaning to all events and actions.
- Present experiences are seen as the consequences of deeds done in the past that must be endured; but no fatalism here, for choices made in the present give shape to the future, either in this life or the next.
- Karma and rebirth are responses to the question patients are prone to ask: "why me?" Anything accidental or unexpected, for which there is no apparent explanation is usually attributed to the unseen hand of karma. Ordinarily Indians do not dwell on karma, and do the best they can. "More commonly when things don't turn out as expected, karma is invoked as an explanation. Helplessness produced by disease and death is relieved by belief in the accumulation of past deeds."[16]
- A major determinant in the response to death is age. No matter how good the medical intervention, sooner or later we must all go. "For death is a certainty for him who has been born and birth is a certainty for him who has died. Therefore, for what is unavoidable, thou shouldest not grieve."[17]
- Only untimely death is profoundly mourned.
- Quality of life is prized more than length of days. Death is preferable to distress and decreptitude.

- A good death is one that happens in the home, and over which a person has control.
- Death is a social event, not merely personal. The extended family comes together to express its collective love and grief while the patient is alive, and continues to participate in the event, through ritual devotion, after the person has died.
- The dead are cremated because fire purifies and "returns bodies to their original form." Children are already considered pure and therefore are not cremated, as in the case of those who live holy lives in the forest.

ĀYURVEDA ON DEATH WITH DIGNITY

Caraka provides a careful analysis of the signs of life and death in the section on *Indriyasthānam.* He makes a division between untimely death, caused by accident or disease, prior to the end of the life span, and timely death that comes at the end, and cannot be indefinitely postponed, because it is natural for all finite beings to die. Just as it is natural for a ripe fruit to release itself from its bonds, so also the end is inevitable for one whose life span is spent, and not even the wisest of *vaidyas* can turn back the hands of time. The role of the doctor is to look for signs indicating death of the moribund person, which Caraka describes in twelve chapters. He follows this with a summary:

> —the vital breath is afflicted, understanding is obstructed, organs discharge strength, activities recede, senses are lost, consciousness is isolated, restlessness and fear enter into the mind, memory and intellect leave, modesty and grace get away, disorders aggravate, ojas and lustre are lost, shadows and shades get deranged, semen flows down, vāyu takes abnormal course, muscle and blood get wasted, the types of agni disappear, joints get dislocated, smells get affected, complexion and voice get deranged, the body is dried up, head acquires fume and cow-dung-like powder, all the pulsating parts of the body get stiffened and devoid of pulsation, the qualities of body parts such as coldness, hotness, softness, hardness etc. change with contrariety, nails get flowered, teeth get muddened, eyelashes get matted, lines appear in head, drugs do not become available as desired, even if obtained they prove ineffective, many difficult diseases having various origins and remedies arise quickly by destroying the strength and ojas: during the course of treatment, inauspicious sound, touch, taste, vision, smell, activity and thoughts arise, fierce dreams appear, disposition of the patient changes on evil side, messengers show adverse signs, features of the dead come forth, normalcy goes

> down fast while morbidity advances, all the portentious signs indicating death are observed. These are the signs of the moribund persons which have been said as proposed and accepted in tradition.[18]

The physician, though observing the signs of death, "should not disclose the approaching death without having been requested for. Even on request, he should not express it if it is liable to cause patient's death or affliction to somemebody else." In the Hindu ethos, death and dying are a family affair. The attending physician is very sensitive to this situation in handling information pertaining to the patient's condition. "The will may be sapped by a physician's declaration of helplessness. A physician usually asks the family to call to the bedside 'all those who need to be present.' The impending death is not explicitly pronounced because words have power. Naming death may invite it too quickly."[19]

Moreover, when death is imminent, "the experienced physician . . . should not be inclined to treat him after observing the fatal signs." The medical manuals classify diseases as "curable" and "incurable," with the instruction that the physician should not waste resources on the treatment of those diseases that fall into the latter category. Once there is a clear manifestation of fatal signs, *all extraordinary means are prohibited on medical and moral grounds*. This decision is bolstered by considerations of professional interest, because "the physican treating an incurable disease certainly suffers from the loss of wealth, learning and reputation and from censure and unpopularity."[20]

Commenting on this situation from the perspective of a physician, Desai says that "it is difficult to imagine a controverys either between ethicist and physician or between family and physician on an issue like 'Do not resuscitate' orders." He acknowledges that modern technology is not as available in India as in the United States, but this factor alone does not sufficiently explain the absence of controversy. "The Hindu is generally allowed to die peacefully, for artificially or mechanically sustained life is held to be of little value. Most people prefer to die in their own beds."[21]

Desai's remarks suggest that Hindu bioethics may have a role to play toward helping Western medicine reconsider its goals and values, especially in the care of the dying. When physicians take the Hippocratic Oath upon receiving their medical degrees, they commit themselves to two fundamental values of medicine: to *prolong life* and to *minimize pain and suffering*. It does not take too many years of practice for the young doctor to discover that these benign principles can fiercely lock horns with one another in a literal life and death struggle.

Timothy E. Quill, a leading physician in the "Death and Dignity" movement, speaks from experience:

> Modern medical treatment has a powerful potential to extend life, yet this same intervention sometimes unintentionally contributes to increased pain and suffering prior to death. Medicine's remarkable success in treating some diseases have led many in our society to value the prolongation of life no matter what the personal consequences, while inadvertently minimizing the increase in human suffering that is often a byproduct. Rather than extending *meaningful* human life, as the Hippocratic Oath intends, medical interventions sometimes result in the prolongation of a painful death. The power and potential of medical technology to produce such diametrically opposed effects should be exercised with the utmost care and restraint.[22]

For its part, Hindu bioethics holds to the position that no person may morally hasten his or her own death or the death of another person by direct means; neither is the individual under any obligation to resist the natural and inevitable approach of death as though it were the enemy of life. Once ordinary means of treatment have failed, and the person chooses to accept the end and prepares for the last steps of life's journey, it becomes medical meddling for the doctor to prolong the dying proces by heroic means. In this context the mandate of *ahiṁsā* for the physician goes beyond the old command: "*Thou shalt not kill,*" to a new command: "*Thou shalt not strive intrusively to keep alive.*"[23]

NOTES

INTRODUCTION

1. Joseph Fletcher, *Humanhood: Essays in Biomedical Ethics* (New York: Prometheus Books, 1979), p. 1.
2. Daniel Callahan, "Biomedical Ethics Today," *Update*, Vol. 1, Number 4, 1985, p. 3.
3. K. Danner Clouser, "Bioethics," in *Encyclopedia of Bioethics*, W. T. Reich, ed. (4 Vols.; New York: The Free Press, 1978), Vol. 1, p. 116.
4. Quoted in Gordon M. Goldstein, "In a Changing World, a New Dawn for Ethics," *New York Times*, April 11, 1993.
5. Jack W. Provonsha, "Religion and the Bioethical Enterprise," *Update*, Vol. 2, Number 1, 1986, p. 2.
6. Kenneth L. Vaux, "Topics at the Interface of of Medicine and Theology," *Health/Medicine and the Faith Traditions*, Martin E. Marty and Kenneth L. Vaux, eds. (Philadelphia: Fortress Press, 1982), pp. 185–215.
7. Seymour Siegel, "Bioethics and Judaism," *Sinai*, Sept. 1987, p. 5.
8. Prakash N. Desai, *Health and Medicine in the Hindu Tradition* (New York: Crossroad, 1989), p. 66.
9. Ibid.
10. Damien Keown, *Buddhism and Bioethics* (New York: St. Martin's Press, 1995), p. ix.

CHAPTER 1. HINDU ETHICS

1. K. N. Upadhyaya, "Dharma as a Regulative Principle," p. 1 (unpublished paper).
2. Kaṭha Up. 2.24 in Robert E. Hume, trans. *The Thirteen Principal Upanishads*, 2d. revised ed. (London: Oxford University Press, 1971), p. 350.
3. Sribhasya IV.1.13.
4. S. K. Saksena, "Philosophical Theories and the Affairs of Men," *The Indian Mind*, Charles E. Moore, ed. (Honolulu: East-West Center Press, 1967), pp. 33,34.
5. S. K. Maitra, *The Ethics of the Hindus* (Calcutta: Calcutta University Press, 1925), p. 1.
6. R. V. X. CXVII.5

7. A. L. Basham, *The Wonder That Was India* (New York: Grove Press, 1954), p. 171.
8. S. K. Saksena, *Essays on Indian Philosophy* (Honolulu: University of Hawaii Press, 1970), p. 40.
9. Manu IV.176.
10. Ibid. II.12.
11. Brh. Up. 2.4.1–3.
12. A. L. Basham, *Aspects of Ancient Indian Culture* (New York: Asia Publishing House, 1970), p. 6.
13. M. K. Gandhi, *Young India*, Sept. 22, 1927.
14. Mbh. III. CLXXX.2.25.
15. K. N. Upadhyaya, *Early Buddhism and the Bhagvadgītā* (Delhi: Motilal Banarsidass, 1971), p. 507.
16. Maitra, op. cit., p. 18.
17. Manu.
18. Maitra, op. cit., p. 5.
19. BG V.25 in *The Bhagvadgītā*, S. Radhakrishnan, trans. (London: George Allen and Unwin Ltd, 1948), p. 184.
20. BG II.34.
21. BG IV.21–22.
22. M. Hiriyanna, *Outlines of Indian Philosophy* (London: Allen and Unwin Ltd, 1970), p. 121.
23. BG II.47.
24. Hiriyanna, loc. cit.
25. M. K. Gandhi, *Young India*, May 27, 1926, p. 189.
26. Chandogya Up. III.17.4.
27. Yoga Sutras II.31.
28. M. K. Gandhi, *Harijan*, January 30, 1937.
29. M. K. Gandhi, *Young India*, June 8, 1921.
30. M. K. Gandhi, *From Yervada Mandir*, 2d. ed. (Amhedabad: Nava Jivan Press, 1935), p. 13.
31. Tom L. Beauchamp, "Ethical Theory," *Contemporary Issues in Bioethics*, Tom L. Beauchamp and LeRoy Walters, eds. (Belmont, Calif.:Wadsworth Publishing Company, 1978), p. 2.
32. Bimal K. Matilal, "Moral Dilemmas: Insights from Indian Epics," in *Moral Dilemmas in the Mahābhārata*, B. K. Matilal, ed. (New Delhi: Motilal Banarsidass, 1989), p. 8.
33. Ibid.
34. Ibid., p. 9.
35. Ibid.
36. Ibid.
37. Ibid. Mbh. Santi. 34.16–32; 109.13–15; 141.39; 142.9.
38. Manu II.11–21.
39. M. Hiriyanna, *Popular Essays in Indian Philosophy* (Mysore: Kavyalaya Publishers, 1952), p. 14.

CHAPTER 2. INDIAN MEDICINE

1. A. L. Basham, "The Practice of Medicine in Ancient and Medieval India," *Asian Medical Systems: A Comparative Study,* Charles Leslie, ed. (Berkeley: University of California Press, 1976), p. 18.
2. Jean Filliozat, *The Classical Doctrine of Indian Medicine* (Delhi: Munshiram Manoharlal, 1964), pp. 86–87.
3. R. V. X. 97.6
4. Henry R. Zimmer, *Hindu Medicine* (Baltimore: The Johns Hopkins Press, 1948), p. 9 ff.
5. Kenneth G. Zysk, *Asceticism and Healing in Ancient India* (New York: Oxford University Press, 1991), vide chapters 1, 2.
6. Ibid., p. 33.
7. Ibid.
8. Ibid.
9. Ibid., p. 118.
10. Basham, *Asian,* op cit., p. 20.
11. J. Filliozat, *The Classical Doctrine of Indian Medicine* (Delhi: Munshiram Manoharlal, 1964), p. 2.
12. *Caraka Saṃhitā,* Priyavrat Sharma, ed./trans. (3 Vols; Varanasi: Chaukhamba Orientalia, 1981), Vol. 1, Su. 1.15–17.
13. Ibid., Introduction, v.
14. Based on CS Su 1.4–31.
15. CS 30.31.
16. Priyadaranjan Ray and Hirendra Nath Gupta, *Caraka Saṃhitā* (Delhi: National Institute of Sciences of India, 1965), p. 3
17. CS Su 30.32. Following translations of P. Ray and H. N. Gupta, *Caraka Saṃhitā,* p. 4.
18. CS Su 30.35.
19. P. Ray, H. N. Gupta, M. Roy, *Suśruta Saṃhitā* (Delhi: Indian National Science Academy, 1980), p. 4.
20. SS Su 1.14–15.
21. Ray et al., *Suśruta,* op. cit., p. 5. Following translation of of P. Ray, H. N. Gupta and M. Roy.
22. Kaviraj Kunjalal Bhishagratna, trans., *Suśruta Saṃhitā,* 3 Vols. (Varanasi: Chowkhamba Sanskrit Series Office, 1991), Vol. 1, p. xv.
23. K. R. Srikantha Murthy, trans. *Vāgbhaṭa's Aṣṭāṅga Hṛdayam* (Varanasi Chowkhabma Sanskrit Series Office, 1991), Vol. 1, p. ix.
24. Ibid., pp. ix–x. Following Murthy, Introduction.
25. Vide Zimmer, op. cit., p. 51.
26. Basham "Asian," op. cit., p. 21.
27. Vide P. V. Sharma, op. cit., vol. 1, p. xxvii.
28. P. Ray, "Caraka," op. cit., p. 5.
29. CS Su. 30.23–24.
30. CS Su. xxx.24–25. Following Priyavrat Sharma translation.

31. P. V. Sharma, "Caraka Oration," delivered at XIIth All India Conference of NIMA, Varanasi, Oct. 23, 1983, p. 7.
32. P. Ray, *Suśruta*, op. cit., p. 2.
33. Surendranath Dasgupta, *A History of Indian Philosophy*, 2 Vols (Cambridge: Cambridge University Press, 1968), Vol. II, p. 273.
34. Ibid.
35. K. N. Udupa, "The Philosophical Basis of Indian Medicine," *Science and Philosophy of Indian Medicine* , K. N. Udupa and R. H. Singh, eds. (Varanasi: Banaras Hindu University, 1990), p. 19.
36. Gerald J. Larson, "Āyurveda and the Hindu Philosophical System," *Self as Body in Asian Theory and Practice,* T. P. Kasulis, R. T. Ames, W. Dissanayake, eds. (New York: State University of New York Press, 1993), p. 109.
37. CS Su. I.42.
38. Kaṭha Up. III.3 ff.
39. Following terminology of P. V. Sharma, op. cit., p. 7.
40. Following Larson's rendition, ibid., p. 108.
41. Ibid., 117.
42. The *Yoga Sutras* of Patanjali I.15 (among other references).
43. Ibid., II.29ff
44. Vide Vasant Lad, *Āyurveda: The Science of Self-Healing* (New Mexico: Lotus Press, 1984), pp. 115–122.
45. Ibid., p. 113.
46. Michael G. Weiss, "Caraka Saṃhitā on the Doctrine of Karma," p. 90 (source unknown).
47. CS Sa.II.44
48. CS Vi. III.29–32
49. CS Vi. III.36 in Weiss translation, ibid., pp. 95–96.
50. CS. Vi. III.38 in Weiss translation.
51. Weiss, ibid., p. 95.
52. Dasgupta, ibid., p. 403.
53. Ibid., p. 404.
54. CS. Su. VIII.30–33.
55. CS Su. XI.3.
56. Ibid. vs. 4.
57. Ibid. vs.5.
58. Ibid. vs. 6.
59. Ibid. vs. 7.
60. Lad, ibid., p. 29.
61. B. Dash and M. M. Junius, *A Handbook of Āyurveda* (Delhi: Concept Publishing Company, 1983), p. 27
62. Ibid., p. 31.
63. Vide Basham, op. cit., p. 18.
64. CS Su. XXIX.5.
65. Ibid. 10–13.
66. CS Su. I.126–133.
67. CS Su. XI.I.

68. SS Su. 11.4.
69. CS Vi. VIII.8
70. CS Vi. VIII.13.
71. SS Su. 11.5.
72. A. Menon and H. F. Habermas, trans., "Oath of Initiation," *Caraka Saṃhitā* in *Cross Cultural Perspectives in Medical Ethics:Readings*, Robert M Veatch, ed. (Boston: Jones and Bartlett Publishers, 1989), pp. 130–132.
73. K. R. Srikanta Murthy, "Professional Ethics in Ancient India," in Veatch, ibid., p. 127.
74. Zimmer, op. cit., p. 76.
75. Murthy, op. cit., p. 128.
76. CS Su IX
77. Ibid. vs. 3.
78. Ibid., vs. 6.
79. Ibid. vs. 13.
80. Ibid. vs. 21.
81. Ibid. vs. 26.
82. Ibid. vs. 7
83. Ibid. vs. 8.
84. Ibid. vs. 9.
85. SS Su X.2.
86. SS Su X.3
87. SS Su XXV.23.
88. SS Su X.1
89. CS Su XXX.29.
90. Basham, Asian, op. cit., p. 33.
91. CS Su XII.13; Su. 29.12.
92. CS Sa IV. 34–40.
93. CS Su VI.27–32.
94. CS Sa III.6–7.
95. Vi. III.4–7
96. CS Su XXV.33
97. Ibid. vs. 36.
98. Ibid.
99. Ibid.
100. Ibid. vs. 38–40
101. Vi. I.24 ff
102. Vi. 11.9.
103. CS Su. XXI.3
104. Ibid. 3–9.
105. Ibid. 4.
106. Ibid.
107. Ibid. vss. 3–9.
108. Ibid. vs. 10.
109. Ibid. vs. 17.
110. Ibid. vs. 10.

111. Ibid. vs. 15.
112. Ibid. vss.10–15.
113. Ibid. vss. 18–19.
114. Ibid. vs. 20.
115. Ibid. vss. 29–34.
116. Ibid. vss. 36–38.
117. Ibid. vss. 39–43
118. Ibid. vss. 52–54.
119. Ibid. vss. 58–59.
120. Sudhir Kakar, "Health and Medicine in the Living Traditions of Hinduism," *Healing and Restoring*, Lawrence E. Sullivan, ed. (New York: Macmillan, 1989), p. 117.
121. Ibid., p. 118.
122. Vi. VI.5–7.
123. CS Sa. I.130–135.
124. Kakar, op cit., p. 120.
125. Ibid., 120–121.
126. CS Su. VIII.17.
127. Ibid. vss. 17–18.
128. Ibid. vs. 19.
129. Ibid.
130. Ibid. vs. 22.
131. Ibid.
132. Ibid.
133. Ibid.
134. Ibid
135. G. P. Dubey, "Preventive Medicine and Personal Hygiene," *Science and Philosophy of Indian Medicine*, op. cit., pp. 99–100.
136. R. H. Singh, "Rasāyana and Vājīkaraṇa," *History of Medicine in India* (Delhi: Indian National Science Academy, 1992), pp. 354–355.
137. CS Ci. I.7–8.
138. SS Ci. XXVII.I
139. Vaidya H. S. Kasture, *Concept of Āyurveda for Perfect Health and Longevity* (Nagpur: Shree Baidyanath Āyurveda Bhavan Private Ltd, 1991), p. 192.
140. CS Ci. I.36–38.
141. Ibid. vs. 16
142. Ibid. vss. 16–24.
143. Ibid. vvs. 29 ff.
144. Singh, op. cit., p. 359.
145. CS Ci. I. 9–12.
146. CS Ci. II.3.
147. CS Ci. II.4–7.
148. CS Ci. II.38–41
149. Ibid. vss. 36–45.
150. Ibid. vss. 30–31

151. CS Vi. III.6 ff.
152. Ibid. vss. 1–7
153. Ibid. vs. 8.
154. *Honolulu Star Bulletin,* Nov. 30, 1998.
155. Ibid.
156. AH Su 1.19–21, in Murthy translation, op. cit.
157. Ibid., p. 12.
158. SS Su. XXIV.2.
159. SS Su. X.6.
160. SS Su. XXIV.4
161. SS Su. ibid. 4–8.
162. SS Su. XXXV.13–14.
163. Ray, *Suśruta,* op. cit., p. 48.
164. Vaidya Shriram Sharma, "Āyurveda: The Science of Life, A Guide to Perfect Health and Longevity," unpublished paper delivered at the University of Hawaii, Honolulu, April 12, 1993.
165. Ibid.

CHAPTER 3. HINDU BIOETHICAL ANALYSIS OF HEALTH/DISEASE AND PHYSICIAN/PATIENT RELATIONSHIPS IN AMERICAN SOCIETY

1. *Caring and Curing,* R. L. Numbers and D. W. Amundsen, eds. (Baltimore: The Johns Hopkins University Press, 1986), p. 360.
2. A. L. Caplan, "The Concepts of Health and Disease," *Medical Ethics,* Robert M. Veatch, ed. (Boston: Jones and Bartlett Publishers, 1989), p. 51.
3. Ibid., p. 52.
4. Ibid., p. 50.
5. Charles Boorse, "On the Distinction Between Disease and Illness," *Philosophy and Public Affairs* 5 (1975): 49–68; cited in Caplan, ibid.
6. Ibid., p. 56.
7. Ibid., p. 56.
8. John Janzen, "Central and Southern African Traditions," *Healing and Restoring,* op. cit., p. 230.
9. Ibid., pp. 229, 230.
10. Ibid., p. 230.
11. Caplan, op. cit., p. 58.
12. *Caring,* op. cit., p. 70.
13. Caplan, op. cit., p. 59.
14. *Medical Ethics,* op. cit., p. 60.
15. Ibid., p. 60.
16. Robert M. Veatch, "Models for Ethical Medicine in a Revolutionary Age," *Ethical Issues in Professional Life,* Joan C. Callahan, ed. (New York: Oxford University Press, 1988), p. 89.
17. Ibid.

18. *Principles of Biomedical Ethics*, Tom L. Beauchamp and James F. Childress, eds. (2d ed.; New York: Oxford University Press, 1994), p. 272.
19. Ibid., p. 274.
20. Ibid., pp. 273, 274.
21. CS Ind. XII. 62–63.
22. Edmund Pellegrino and David Thomasma, "For the Patient's Good: The Restoration of Beneficence in Health Care" (New York: Oxford University Press, 1988), pp. 25, 32; cited in *Principles of Biomedical Ethics*, Tom Beauchamp and James Childress, eds. (New York: Oxford University Press, 1994), pp. 72, 73.
23. Ibid., p. 91.
24. Ibid.
25. Ibid.
26. Howard Brody, "The Physician/Patient Relationship," *Medical Ethics*, op. cit., p. 72.
27. CS Su. IX.1ff.
28. Ibid. vs. 3.
29. Ibid. vss. 6–9.
30. Ibid. vs. 9.
31. CS Vi. VIII.13.
32. CS Su. IX.13.
33. CS Vi. VIII.13.
34. Ibid.
35. Ibid.
36. See "Oath of Initiation."

CHAPTER 4. TECHNOLOGY AND THE WOMB

1. *Time*, March 23, 1987.
2. Manu IX.96, *The Sacred Books of the East*, F. Max Muller, ed. (Motilal Banarsidass: Delhi, 1984), Vol. XXV, p. 344.
3. Mbh. XII, 34.14; III, 200.4 f.
4. Gautama, XVIII.4–5.
5. Ibid. vs. 14.
6. Manu IX. 59–60.
7. Mbh. I, 120 ff. Vide Johann J. Meyer, *Sexual Life in Ancient India* (New York: Dorset Press, 1995), p. 163.
8. Manu IX.32.
9. Basham, *Wonder*, op. cit., p. 174.
10. Desai, op. cit., p. 67.
11. Ibid., p. 68.
12. Richard A. McCormick, *How Brave a New World* (Washington: Georgetown University Press, 1981), see chapter 16.
13. Desai, op. cit., p. 68.
14. I, 105. 1–2, in Meyer, op. cit., p. 161.

CHAPTER 5. DILEMMAS AT BIRTH

1. *New England Journal of Medicine*, September 1994; see related report: "'Miracle babies' have problems down the road," *Associated Press*, Sept. 1994.
2. Quoted in Dick Thompson, "Should Every Baby Be Saved?," *Time*, June 11, 1990.
3. Ibid.
4. Claudia Wallis, "Baby Fae Loses Her Battle," *Time*, November 26, 1984.
5. "Baby Conceived to Save a Life Gets Her Chance," *Star-Bulletin*, June 4, 1991.

CHAPTER 6. WHEN PARENTS LET CHILDREN SUFFER FOR REASONS OF FAITH

1. Mary Baker Eddy, *Science and Health with Key to the Scriptures* (Boston: The First Church of Christ Scientist, 1971), p. 429.
2. RV V.4.10.
3. SS Sa 111.12.
4. Rajbali Pandey, *Hindu Saṁskāras* (Delhi: Motilal Banarsidass, 1991), p. 34.
5. Terence F. Ackerman, "The Limits of Beneficence: Jehovah's Witnesses and Childhood Cancer," *The Hastings Center Report*, Vol. 10, Number 4, August 1980, p. 14.
6. R. N. Dandekar, "The Role of Man in Hinduism," *The Religion of the Hindus*, Kenneth W. Morgan, ed. (New York: Ronald Press, 1953), p. 138.
7. Taitt. Up. 1.11.1–4 in Hume, op. cit.
8. Ackerman, op cit., p. 15.
9. "Convention on the Rights of the Child," *Religious Dimensions of Child and Family Life*, Harold Coward and Philip Cooke, eds. (Victoria: Centre for Studies in Religion and Society, 1996), pp. 174, 175.

CHAPTER 7. THE ETHICS OF CONTRACEPTION

1. Family Planning Perspective, January, February 1998; a study sponsored by Alan Guttmacher Institute; researched by Stan K. Henshaw; in *Honolulu Star-Bulletin*, Feb. 28, 1998.
2. Richard P. McBrien, ed., *Catholicism* (Minneapolis: Winston Press, 1970), p. 1016.
3. Ibid.
4. Brh. Up. VI.4.10 in Hume, op. cit.
5. Seshagiri Rao, "Population Ethics: A Hindu Perspective," *Encyclopedia of Bioethics*, vol. 3, op. cit., p. 1271.

CHAPTER 8. THE ETHICS OF PRENATAL DIAGNOSIS FOR SEX SELECTION

1. Seema Sirohi, "Indians Embrace the 'Boy-Girl Test,' Associated Press, in *Honolulu Star-Bulletin*, March 22, 1988.
2. Ibid.
3. Sundari Nanda, quoted in "Dowry Deaths Multiply in India," *Washington Post*, in *The Honolulu Advertiser*, April 16, 1995.
4. Ibid.
5. 12/10/1999.
6. *UNDP's Human Development Report*, 1999; supplied by Dr. Krishna Jafa, The Population Institute, Washington, D. C.

CHAPTER 9. THE ETHICS OF THE HUMAN GENOME PROJECT

1. Leon Jaroff, "Seeking a Godlike Power," *Time*, Fall, 1992, p. 58.
2. Mark Skolnick, quoted in Jaroff, ibid.
3. Dick Thompson, "The Gene Machine," *Time*, January 24, 2000.
4. Gītā, 2.18.
5. Vide Sharon J. Durfy and Amy E. Grotevant, "The Human Genome Project," *National Reference Center for Bioethical Literature*, Kennedy Institute of Ethics, Georgetown University, Washington, DC, December 1991, p. 3.

CHAPTER 10. THE ETHICS OF GENETIC ENGINEERING

1. W. French Anderson, "A Cure That May Cost Us Ourselves," *Newsweek*, Jan. 3, 2000.
2. R. Michael Blaese, "Gene Therapy, the Science Beyond the Story," speech delivered at the East-West Center, Honolulu, Feb. 22, 1999.
3. Quoted by Helen Altonn, "Doctors Map Out Genetic Treatments," *Honolulu Star-Bulletin*, Feb. 20, 1999.
4. Mary Carrington Coutts, "Human Gene Therapy," *Scope Note 24, National Reference Center for Bioethics Literature*, Kennedy Institute of Ethics, Georgetown University, Washington, DC, p. 4.
5. In Angie Cannon, "Humility at the Frontier," *U. S. News and World Report*, Dec. 20, 1999, p. 60.
6. W. French Anderson, "Genetics and Human Malleability," *Moral Issues and Christian Response*, Paul T. Jersild and Dale A. Johnson, eds. (Fortworth: Harcourt Brace College Publishers, 1993), p. 308.
7. *Nature*, Sept. 1999.
8. In Michael D. Lemonick, "Smart Genes?," *Time*, September 13, 1999
9. In Nancy Gibbs, "If We Have It, Do We Use It?," *Time*, ibid.

10. The Bhagavadgītā, VI.5. in Radhakrishnan translation, op. cit.
11. Anderson, "Malleability," op. cit., p. 309.
12. Ibid.
13. In Gibbs, op. cit., p. 59.
14. Ibid.
15. Harold Coward, "Ethics and Genetic Engineering in Indian Philosophy," unpublished paper presented at the *Eighth East-West Philosophers' Conference*, University of Hawaii, Jan. 19, 2000.
16. Seshagiri Rao, "Mahatama Gandhi and Reformation of Hinduism," *In Search of Hinduism*, Cromwell Crawford, ed. (New York: Unification Theological Seminary, 1986), p. 156.

CHAPTER 11. THE ETHICS OF CLONING

1. In Jeffrey Kluger, "Will We Follow The Sheep," *Time*, March 10, 1997.
2. Daniel Callahan, "Cloning: The Work Not Done," *Hastings Report*, Sept.-Oct., 1997.
3. "Playing God," *Hinduism Today*, June 1997, p. 24ff.
4. Francis Collins, "Science and Faith," *Context*, May 15, 2000.
5. "Playing God," loc. cit.

CHAPTER 12. THE ETHICS OF POPULATION GROWTH

1. "Explosive Growth Defines 20th Century," *Popline*, May–June 1999, p. 4.
2. "World Population Reaches Six Billion," *Popline*, Sept.-Oct. 1999.
3. Ibid.
4. Genaro C. Armas, "India, Africa to Set the Pace," Associated Press, in *Honolulu Star-Bulletin*, June 8, 2000, p. A-12.
5. Ibid.
6. Fornos quoted in "India Lacks Political Commitment to Family Planning," *MID-DAY*, Dec. 8, 1999, p. 6.
7. Wadia quoted in Archana Sharma, "Number Cruncher," ibid.
8. CS Sa. VIII.3–7.
9. US AID's International Population and Family Planning Assistance, in "Appendix," *The Population Institute Manual*, Washington, DC, May 1999.
10. Ibid.
11. Ibid.
12. Ibid.
13. Singh quoted in "From Bucharest to Cairo: Population Stabilization Deliberations," *Toward the 21st Century, The Population Institute*, Number 4, 1994.
14. Fornos, op. cit.
15. Kishor quoted in Armas, op. cit.
16. Fornos, op. cit.

17. *Human Development Report 1999*, courtesy of Dr. Krishna Jafa, *The Population Institute*, op. cit.
18. RV. x.85, 42–45.
19. Manu 9.137–138.
20. Ibid.
21. Ibid.

CHAPTER 13. THE ETHICS OF AGING: MAXIMIZING THE QUALITY OF LATER LIFE

1. *Time*, March 6, 1995.
2. Patrice A. Cruise, "The Booming Elderly Population: The Economic Crunch and Generational Equity," *Update*, vol. 10, no. 2, 1994, p. 2.
3. Ibid.
4. "Aging: New Answers to Old Questions," *National Geographic*, Nov. 1997, p. 11.
5. Ibid.
6. Christopher Lasch, "Aging in a Culture without a Future," *Hastings Center Report*, vol. 7, no. 4, Aug. 1977, p. 42.
7. Ibid.
8. Joel Kurtzman and Philip Gordon, *No More Dying: The Conquest of Aging and the Extension of Human Life* (Los Angeles: J. P. Tarcher, Inc., 1976); Albert Rosenfeld, *Prolongevity* (New York: Alfred A. Knopf, 1976).
9. Lasch, op. cit., p. 42.
10. Quoted in Lasch, ibid.
11. John W. Rowe and Robert L. Kahn, *Successful Aging* (New York: Pantheon Books, 1998), pp. xii, xiii.
12. Ibid., p. xi.
13. Ibid., p. 38.
14. Ibid., p. 40.
15. Ibid., p. 42.
16. Ibid., p. xii.
17. Ibid., p. 46.
18. Lasch, op. cit., p. 43.
19. Kevin O'Hanlon, "Abuse and Neglect of Elderly," Associated Press in *Honolulu Star-Bulletin*, Nov. 15, 1997.
20. "How Medicine Mistreats the Elderly," *U. S. News and World Report*, Jan. 18, 1993.
21. "Aging Athletes: Keep On Keeping On," *Harvard Health Letter*, March, 1977.
22. Lasch, loc. cit.
23. Lasch, loc. cit.
24. Laws of Manu VI. 1ff.
25. Drew Leder, "The Trouble with Successful Aging," *Parkridge Center Bulletin*, no. 6, Oct./Nov. 1998.

26. Ibid.
27. Shrinivas Tilak, *Religion and Aging in the Indian Tradition* (New York: State University of New York Press, 1989), vide Foreword.

CHAPTER 14. THE ETHICS OF DEATH AND DYING

1. Sylvia Vatuk, "The Art of Dying in Hindu India," in *Facing Death*, ed. Howard M. Spiro, Mary G. McCrea (New Haven: Yale University Press, 1996), p. 121.
2. David Landy, "Death: An Anthropological Perspective," in Death, *Reich*, op. cit., vol. 1, 228.
3. Anantanand Rambachan, "Hinduism," *Life After Death in World Religions*, ed. Harold Coward (New York: Orbis Books, 1997), p. 66 ff.
4. Kaṭha Up. 3.7 in Hume, op. cit.
5. Bṛhadāraṇyaka Up. 4.4.2.
6. Bhagavadgītā 9.25.
7. Kaṭha Up. 6.16.
8. Bhagavadgītā 9.25.
9. Ibid., 1.40–42.
10. Sarvepalli Radhakrishnan, *Selected Writings on Philosophy and Culture*, ed. Robert A. McDermott (New York: Dutton, 1970).
11. Frank E. Reynolds, "Death: Eastern Thought," in Reich, op. cit. vol. 1, p. 232.
12. Bṛhadāraṇyaka Up. 1.3.28.
13. Kaṭha Up. 6.14.
14. Muṇḍaka Up. 3.2.8–9.
15. Kakar, op. cit., p. 32.
16. Desai, op. cit., p. 32.
17. Bhagavadgītā 2.27.
18. CS Indriya. XII. 43–46.
19. Desai, op. cit., p. 94.
20. CS Su. I.X. 7–8.
21. Desai, op. cit., p. 94.
22. Thomas E. Quill, *Death and Dignity* (New York: W. W. Norton and Company, 1993), p. 43.
23. Vide Arthur Hugh Clough in Thomas A. Wassmer, "Ethical and Moral Issues Involved in Recent Medical Advances," *Villanova Law Review*, vol. 13, no. 4, p. 732, 1968.

GLOSSARY

acit—matter, material
advaita—monism
Agni—god of fire
ahaṅkāra—ego
ahiṁsā—nonviolence
amṛtya—immortality
anārabdha—karma that has not begun to bear fruit
araṇya—the forest
artha—worldly prosperity; one of four human ends
asat—unreal
āśrama—stage of life
Atharvaveda—the fourth veda
atithis—chance guests
ātma-ghata—self-killing
ātma-hatyā—self-killing
ātman—the self
avidyā—original ignorance
Āyurveda—the science of longevity
bala—strength
Bhagavadgītā—The Lord's Song; a part of the Mahābhārata
bhrūṇa-hatyā—feticide
Brahmacarya—the stage of the religious student
Brahman—Ultimate Reality
Brāhmaṇas—Vedic texts discussing sacrificial rites
buddhi—intelligence, cognition
cit—self
dayā—compassion
dharma duty, law, righteousness
Dharmaśāstras—sacred texts dealing with morality
dīkṣā—consecration ceremony
Ganga—the most sacred river
guṇas—basic properties
hiṁsā—causing pain or killing out of anger
jauhar—rite by which womenfolk of Rajput warriors would collectively immolate themselves to preserve honor
jīva—the individual embodied soul
jivadaya—kindness to creatures
jīvanmukti—the state of self-realization while yet in the body

kāma—pleasures of the five senses; one of four human ends
karma—action; the law of cause and effect in the moral sphere
Mahābhārata—one of India's two great epics; discussions of morals
mahābhūtas—gross elements
mahā-makha—great sacrifice
mahāpātākas—atrocious sins
mahāprasthāna—the Great Journey
Manu—the most eminent Hindu lawgiver; teaches the four stages and ends of life
mokṣa—liberation
niyoga—levirate marriage
pāpa—evil
parināmavāda—theory of causality
parivrājaka—ascetic
Pārvatī—wife of Śiva
piṇḍa—morsel of ritual oblation of food to an ancestor
pitṛ—deceased forefathers, existing in heavenly realms
prajati—parenthood
prakṛti—the material principle
pralaya—state of dissolution
prārabdha karma—karma that has come to fruition
prayopaveśa—fasting
Purāṇas—popular moral stories about legendary gods and heroes
Puruṣa—the Supreme Being; the spiritual principle
puruṣārthas—the four supreme values of life
Rāmāyaṇa—one of India's two great epics; narrating the story of Visnu's incarnation as Rāmā
rati—pleasure
Ṛgveda—first of the four Vedas, composed of hymns; essential for understanding Hindu thought
ṛṇatraya—triad of obligations
ṛta—natural and moral order of the universe
sādhu—a holy man
sakhya—companionship
Śakti—divine Mother; female creative energy
sallekhanā—starving oneself to death
Sāṁkara—eighth-century philosopher of nondualism
Sāṁkhya—a philosophy of dualistic realism
saṁsāra—the wheel of rebirth; the world of impermanence and suffering
saṁskāras—innate tendencies of a person
sañcita karma—karma accumulted from past lives
sannyāsin—one who has abandoned the world and lives the holy life
sapiṇḍa—blood relations
saṛga—state of evolution
satī—a virtuous, devoted widow who immolates herself on the funeral pyre of her husband

sattva—one of the three basic properties, of the nature of truth, purity, and light
satya-rakṣā—protecting the truth
Smṛti—the body of sacred lore remembered and pased on by tradition
śrāddha—ceremony honoring dead ancestors
Śruti—scriptures revealed to ancient rsis, identified with the Vedas
Upaniṣads—ancient philosophic treatises forming final sections of the Vedas
vāhana—the mount of a god
vaidya—a physician
vartamāna-karma—karma generated in present life
Vedānta—a system of philosophy based on the Upaniṣads

BIBLIOGRAPHY

Ahmed, A. F. S. *Social Ideas and Social Change in Bengal, 1818–1835*. Leiden, E. J. Brill, 1965.

Ames, R. T., T. Dissanayake, and P. Kasulis, eds. *Self as Body in Asian Theory and Practice*. New York: State University of New York Press, 1993.

Apte, U. M. *The Sacrament of Marriage in Hindu Society*. Delhi: Ajanta Publications, 1978.

Banerji, S. C. *Indian Society in the Mahābhārata*. Varanasi: Bharata Manisha, 1976.

Basham, A. L. *Aspects of Ancient Indian Culture*. New York: Asia Publishing House, 1970.

———. *The Wonder That Was India*. New York: Grove Press, 1954.

Basu, B. D., ed. *Parthasarathi*. Allahabad: Pāṇini Office, 1924.

Beauchamp, Tom. L. and Leroy Walters, eds. *Contemporary Issues in Bioethics*. Belmont, Calif.: Wadsworth Publishing Company, 1978.

Beauchamp, Tom. L. and Childress, James F., eds. *Principles of Medical Ethics*. New York: Oxford University Press, 1994.

Bethge, Eberhard, ed. *Ethics* by Dietrich Bonhoeffer. New York: Macmillan, 1965.

Bhargava, P. L. *Fundamentals of Hinduism*. Delhi: Munshiram Manoharlal, 1982.

Bhisagrata, Kaviraj Kunjalal, trans. *Suśruta Saṃhitā*, 3 vols. Varanasi: Chowkhamba Sanskrit Series Office, 1991.

Blumenthal, Susan J., and David J. Klupfer, eds. *Suicide Over the Life Cycle: Risk Factors, Assessments, and Treatment of Suicidal Patients*. Washington: American Psychiatric Press, 1990.

Bose, A. C. *Hymns from the Vedas*. Bombay: Asia Publishing House, 1966.

Brown, W. N. *Man in the Universe*. Berkeley: University of California Pres, 1970

Buhler, G. Trans., *The Laws of Manu*, in *Sacred Books of the East*, Vol. XXXV, F. M.Muller, ed. Oxford: Clarendon Press, 1886.

———. Trans., *Vasiṣṭha* and *Baudhāyana*, in *Sacred Books of the East*, Vol. XII, F. M. Muller, ed. Oxford: Clarendon Press, 1879.

———. Trans., *Āpastamba* and *Gautama*, in *Sacred Books of the East*, Vol. I, F. M. Muller, ed. Oxford: Clarendon Press, 1879.

Callahan, Joan, ed. *Ethical Issues in Professional Life*. New York: Oxford University Press, 1988.

Carrington, Mary, ed. *National Reference Centre for Bioethics* Literature. Washington: Georgetown University Press.

Chakravarti, Chandra. *Sex Life in Ancient India*. Calcutta: Firma K. L. Mukhopadhyay, 1963.

Chakravati, Satis Chandra, ed. *The Father of Modern India*. Calcutta: Rammohan Roy Centenary Committee, 1935.

Chatterjee, S. C. and Dutta, D. M., eds. *An Introduction to Indian Philosophy*. Calcutta: University Press, 1968.

Chattopadhyaya, Sudhakar. *Social Life in Ancient India*. Calcutta: Academic Publishers, 1965.

Chopra, Deepak. *Perfect Health*. New York: Harmony Books, 1991.

———. *Ageless Body, Timeless Mind*. New York: Harmony Books, 1993.

———. *Boundless Energy*. New York: Three Rivers Press, 1995.

Coward, Harold and Philip Cooke, eds. *Religious Dimensions of Child and Family*. Victoria: Centre for Studies in Religion and Society, 1996.

Coward, Harold, Lipner, Julius, and Young, Katherine, eds. *Hindu Ethics*. New York: State University of New York Press, 1989.

Coward, Harold, ed. *Life After Death in World Religions*. New York: Orbis Books, 1997.

Crawford, S. Cromwell. *The Evolution of Hindu Ethical Ideals*. Honolulu: The Univesity Press of Hawaii, 1982.

———. *Ram Mohan Roy*. New York: Paragon House, 1987.

———. ed. *World Religions and Global Ethics*. New York: Paragon House, 1989.

———. ed. *In Search of Hinduism*. New York: The Unification Theological Seminary Press, 1986.

———. *Dilemmas of Life and Death:* Hindu Ethics in a North American Context. New York: State University of New York Press, 1995.

Dandekar, Kumudini. *The Elderly in India*. Delhi: Sage Publications, 1996.

Dasgupta, Surendranath. *A History of Indian Philosophy*. 2 vols. Cambridge: Cambridge University Press, 1969.

Dash, B. and Junius, M. M., eds. *A Handbook of Āyurveda*. Delhi: Concept Publishing Co., 1983.

Desai, Prakash, N. *Health and Medicine in the Hindu Tradition*. New York: Crossroad, 1989.

Deutsch, Eliot, trans. *The Bhagavadgītā*. New York: Holt, Rinehart and Winston, 1968.

Dutta, M. N., ed. *The Dharam Shastra: Hindu Religious Codes*. 5 vols. New Delhi: Cosmo Publications, 1979.

Eddy, Mary Baker. *Science and Health, With Key to the Scriptures*. Boston: The First Church of Christ Scientist, 1971.

Eggeling, J.trans. *Satapatha Brāhmaṇa*, in *Sacred Books of the East,* Vols. XII, XXVI, XLI, XLIII, XLIV. F. M. Muller, ed. Oxford: Clarendon Press.

Eliade, Mircea, ed. *The Encyclopedia of Religion*. 12 vols. New York: Macmillan and Free Press, 1987.

Farquhar, J. N. *An Outline of the Religious Literature of India*. Delhi: Motilal Banarsidass, 1984.

Filliozat, Jean. *The Classical Doctrine of Indian Medicine*. Delhi. Manoharlal Munshiram, 1964.

Fletcher, Joseph. *Humanhood: Essays in Biomedical Ethics*. New York: Prometheus Books, 1979.

Garbe, R. "Sankhya," in *Encyclopaedia of Religion and Ethics*. Vol. 11. New York: Scribners, 1925.

Ghosh, J. *Sāṁkhya and Modern Thought*. Calcutta: The Book Company, 1930.

Ghosh, Shyam. *Hindu Concept of Life and Death*. Delhi: Munshiram Manoharlal, 1989.

Hamel, Ron, ed. *Active Euthanasia, Religion, and the Public Debate*. Chicago: The Park Ridge Center, 1991.

Hastings, James, ed. *Encyclopaedia of Religion and Ethics*. Edinburgh: T. and T. Clark, 1980 reprint.

Herring, Basil. *Ethics and Halakah for Our Time: Sources and Commentary*. New York: Ktav Publishing House, 1984.

Hiriyanna, M. *The Essentials of Hindu Philosophy*. London: Allen and Unwin, 1967.

———. *Popular Essays in Indian Philosophy*. Mysore: Kavyalaya Publishers, 1952.

———. *Outlines of Indian Philosophy*. London: Allen and Unwin, 1970.

Hume, R. E., trans. *The Thirteen Principal Upanishads*. 3d. ed. Oxford: Oxford University Press, 1971.

Humphry, Derek. *Final Exit*. Oregon: The Hemlock Society, 1991.

Hutchins, Robert M., ed. *The Great Books of the Western World*. 50 vols. Chicago: Encyclopaedia Britannica, 1952.

Iyer, Raghavan. *The Moral and Political Thought of Mahatama Gandhi*. New York: Oxford University Press, 1973.

Jersild, Paul T. and Dale A. Johnson, eds. *Moral Issues and Christian Response*. Fort Worth: Holt, Rinehart and Winston, 1988.

Jha, G., trans. *Gautama's Nyāyasūtras* (with Vātsyāyana's *Bhāṣya*), in Poona Oriental series, 59. Poona: Poona Book Agency, 1939.

———. *Padārthadharmasaṃgraha of Praśastapāda*. Allahabad: E. J. Lazarus and Co., 1916.

———. The Tattva-Kaumudi. 2d. ed. Poona: Oriental Book Agency, 1934.

———. *The Tattva-Kaumudī* (Vacaspati Misra's Commentary on the *Sāṁkhya-Karika*). 2d. rev. ed. Poona: Oriental Books Agency, 1934.

———. *Pūrva-Mīmāṃsā in its Sources*. Benares: Hindu University Press, 1942.

———. *Mīmāṃsā sūtra*. Baroda: Oriental Institute, 1936.

———. *Ślokavārtika* by Kumarila Bhatta. Calcutta: Asiatic Society of Bengal, 1909.

Jhingran, Saral. *Aspects of Hindu Morality*. Delhi: Motilal Banarsidass, 1989.

Jolly, J. trans. *The Institutes of Vishnu* in the *Sacred Books of the East*, F. M. Muller, ed. Oxford: Oxford University Press, 1880.

Justice, Christopher. *Dying the Good Death: The Pilgrimage to Die in India's Holy City*. New York: State University of New York Press, 1997.

Kakar, Sudhir. *Shamans, Mystics and Doctors*. Boston: Beacon Press, 1982.

Intimate Relations: Exploring India Sexuality. Chicago: University of Chicago Press, 1990.

Kanal, S. P. *Dialogues on Indian Culture*. Delhi: Panchal Press Publications, 1950.

Kane, Pandurang Vaman. *History of Dharmaśāstra*. 6. vols. Poona: Bhandarkar Oriental Research Institute, 1973.

Kasture, H. S. *Concept of Āyurveda for Perfect Health and Longevity*. Nagpur: Shree Baidyanath Āyurveda Bhavan Private Limited. 1991.

Keith, A. B. *Indian Logic and Atomism*. Oxford: Clarendon Press, 1921.

———. *The Religion and Philosophy of the Vedas and Upanishads,* in Harvard Oriental Series. Vol. XXXII, C. R. Lanman, ed. Cambridge, Mass.: Harvard University Press, 1925.

Keown, Damien. *Buddhism and Bioethics*. New York: St. Martin's Press, 1995.

Kurtzman, Joel and Gordon, Philip. *No More Dying: The Conquest of Aging and the Extension of Human Life*. Los Angeles: J. P. Tarcher, Inc., 1976.

———. Lad, Vasant. *Āyurveda: The Science of Self-Healing*. New Mexico: Lotus Press, 1984.

———. *The Complete Book of Ayurvedic Home Remedies*. New York: Harmony Books, 1998.

Lingat, Robert. *The Classical Law of India*. Berkeley: University of California Press, 1973.

Maitra, S. K. *The Ethics of the Hindus*. Calcutta: Calcutta University Press, 1925.

Marty, Martin, E., and Vaux, Kenneth L., eds. *Health Medicine and the Faith Traditions*. Philadelphia: Fortress Press, 1982.

Matilal, B. K., ed. *Moral Dilemmas in the Mahābhārata*. New Delhi: Motilal Banarsidass, 1989.

Maurer, Walter H. *Pinnacles of India's Past*. Philadelphia: John Benjamins Publishing Company, 1986.

Meyer, Johann. *Sexual Life in Ancient India*. New York: Dorset Press, 1995.

Moore, Charles E., ed. *The Indian Mind*. Honolulu: East-West Center Press, 1967.

Morgan, Kenneth W., ed. *The Religion of the Hindus*. New York: Ronald Press, 1953.

Motwani, K. *Manu Dharma Sastra*. Madras: Ganesh and Co., 1958.

Mukhopadhyaya, G. *Studies in the Upaniṣads*. Calcutta: Sanskrit College Series, 1960.

Muller, F. Max. *Six Systems of Indian Philosophy*. London: Longmans, 1928.

———. ed. *Sacred Books of the East*. 50 vols. New Delhi: Motilal Banarsidass, 1987 reprint.

Murthy, K. R. Srikantha. trans. *Vāgbhaṭa's Aṣṭānga Hṛdayam*. Varanasi: Chowkhamba Sanskrit Series Office, 1991.

McBrien, Richard, ed. *Catholicism*. Minneapolis: Winston Press, 1970.

McCormick, Richard A. *How Brave a New World*. Washington: Georgetown University Press, 1981.

McDermott, Robert A. ed. *Selected Writings on Philosophy and Culture*. New York: Dutton, 1970

Nag, Kalidas and Debajyoti Burman, eds. *The English Works of Raja Rammohun Roy*. Calcutta: Sadharan Brahmo Samaj, 1946.

Nikhilananda, Swami. *The Upanishads*. New York: Harper and Row, 1964.

Numbers, R. L. and Amundsen, D. W., eds. *Caring and Curing*. Baltimore: The Johns Hopins University Press, 1986.

Olivelle, Patrick. *Samnyasa Upaniṣads*. New York: Oxford University Press, 1992.

Pandey, Rajbali. *Hindu Saṁskāras*. Delhi: Motilal Banarsidass, 1991.

Prabhu, P. H. *Hindu Social Organization*. Bombay: Popular Prakashan, 1963.

Prasada, R., trans. *Yoga Sutras of Patanjali*, in *Sacred Books of the Hindus*. Vol IV. B. D. Basu, ed. Allahabad: Pāṇini Office, 1924.

Quill, Thomas E. *Death and Dignity*. New York: W. W. Norton and Co., 1993.

Radhakrishnan, S. and Moore, C., eds. *A Sourcebook in Indian Philosophy*. Princeton, N.J.: Princeton University Press, 1967.

Radhakrishnan, Sarvepalli. *The Vedānta*. London: Allen and Unwin, 1928.

———. *Indian Philosophy*. 2 vols. London: Allen and Unwin, 1966.

———. *The Hindu View of Life*. New York: Macmillan, 1965.

———. trans. *The Bhagavadgītā*. London. Allen and Unwin, 1948.

———. trans. *The Brahmā Sūtra*. London: Allen and Unwin, 1960.

Ramaswamy, T. N., trans. *Essentials of Indian Statecraft: Kauṭilya's Arthaśāstra for Contemporary Readers*. Bombay: Asia Publishing House, 1962.

Ray, Priyadaranjan, Hirendranath Gupta, and Mira Roy, eds. *Suśruta Saṃhitā*. Delhi: National Science Academy, 1980.

Ray, Priyadaranjan, and Hirendrnath Gupta, eds. *Caraka Saṃhitā*. Delhi: National Institute of Sciences of India, 1965.

Regan, Tom, ed. *Moral Philosophy: Matters of Life and Death*. New York: Random House, 1980.

Reich, W. T., general ed. *Encyclopedia of Bioethics*. 4 vols. New York: The Free Press, 1978.

Rosenfeld, Albert. *Prolongevity*. New York: Alfred A. Knopf, 1976.

Rowe, John W. and Robert L. Kahn, *Successful Aging*. New York: Pantheon Books, 1998.

Saint Augustine. *City of God*, trans. Gerald G. Walsh et al. New York: Image Books, 1958.

Saksena, S. K. *Essays on Indian Philosophy*. Honolulu: University of Hawaii Press, 1970.

Schneidman, Edwin. *Definitions of Suicide*. New York: John Wiley, 1985.

Sharma, I. C. *Ethical Philosophies of India*. Nebraska: Johnsen Publishing House, 1965.

Sharma, Priyavrat, ed. and trans. *Caraka Saṃhitā*. 3 vols. Varanasi/Delhi: Chaukambha Orientalia, 1981.

———. *History of Medicine in India*. Delhi: Indian National Science Academy, 1992.

Sharma, Shiv. *The System of Āyurveda*. Delhi: Neeraj Publishing House, 1929.

———. *Realms of Āyurveda*. Delhi: Arnold-Heinemann, 1979.

Sheikh, Anees and Katharina S. Sheikh. *Eastern and Western Approaches to Healing: Ancient Wisdom and Modern Knowledge*. New York: John Wiley and Sons, 1989.

Singh, R. H. *Panca Karma Therapy*. Varanasi: Chowkhamba Sanskrit Series Office, 1992.

Singhal, G. D. *Surgical Ethics in Āyurveda*.Varanasi: Chowkhamba Sanskrit Series Office, 1963.

Sinha, N. trans. *The Vaiśeṣika Sūtras of Kaṇāda*, in *Sacred Books of the Hindus*. Vol VI. B. D. Basu, ed. Allahabad: The Pāṇini Office, 1923.

Smart, Ninian. *Worldviews: Crosscultural Explorations of Human Beliefs*. New Jersey: Prentice Hall, 1995.

Spiro, Howard M. and Mary G. McCrea, eds. *Facing Death*. New Haven: Yale University Press, 1996.

Steiner, Gilbert Y., ed. *The Abortion Dispute and the American System*. New York: The Brookings Institute, 1983.

Stutley, Margaret and James Stutley, eds. *Harper's Dictionary of Hinduism*. New York: Harper and Row, 1977.

Sullivan, Lawrence E., ed. *Healing and Restoring*. New York: Macmillan, 1989.

Thadani, N., trans. *Mimansa: The Secret of the Sacred Books of the Hindus*. Delhi: Bharati Research Institute, 1952.

Thibaut, G., trans. *Vedānta-Sūtras (with Rāmānuja's Commentary)* in *Sacred Books of the East*. Vol. XLIII. Delhi: Motilal Banarsidass, 1962.

———. *Vedānta-Sutras (with Śaṇkaras Commentary)* in *Sacred Books of the East*. Vol. XXXIV. Ox:ford: Clarendon Press, 1890.

Tilak, Srinivas. *Religion and Aging in the Indian Tradition*. New York: State University of New York, 1989.

Tirtha, Swami Sada Shiva. *The Āyurveda Encyclopedia*. Bayville, NY: Āyurveda Holistic Center Press, 1998.

Udupa, K. N. and Singh, R. H., eds. *Science and Philosophy of Indian Medicine*. Varanasi: Banaras Hindu University, 1990.

Upadhyaya, K. N. *The Bhagavadgītā and Early Buddhism*. Delhi: Motilal Banarsidass, 1971.

Vaux, Kenneth, L. and Marty, Martin E., eds. *Health/Medicine and The Faith Traditions*. Philadelphia: Fortress Press, 1982.

Veatch, Robert M. ed. *Cross-Cultural Perspectives in Medical Ethics: Readings*. Boston: Jones and Bartlett, 1989.

———. *Medical Ethics*. Boston: Jones and Bartlett Publishers, 1989.

Verma, Vinod. *Āyurveda: A Way of Life*. York Beach, Me: Samuel Weiser, Inc., 1995.

Vidyabhusana, S. C., trans. *The Nyāya Sūtras of Gotama* in *Sacred Books of the Hindus*. Vol VII. B. D. Basu, ed. Allahabad: The Pāṇini Office, 1930.

Weiss, Mitchell. *History of Psychiatry in India*. Cambridge: Harvard Medical School, 1986.

Zimmer, Heinrich. *Hindu Medicine*. Baltimore: The Johns Hopkins Press, 1948.

Zysk, Kenneth. *Asceticism and Healing in Ancient India*. New York: Oxford University Press, 1991.

———. *Religious Medicine: The History and Evolution of Indian Medicine*. New Brunswick: Transaction Publishers, 1993.

INDEX

Printed in the United States
50517LVS00001B/340-438

9 780791 457801